Chas Martin
Massillon
Ohio
Jany 14. 1851

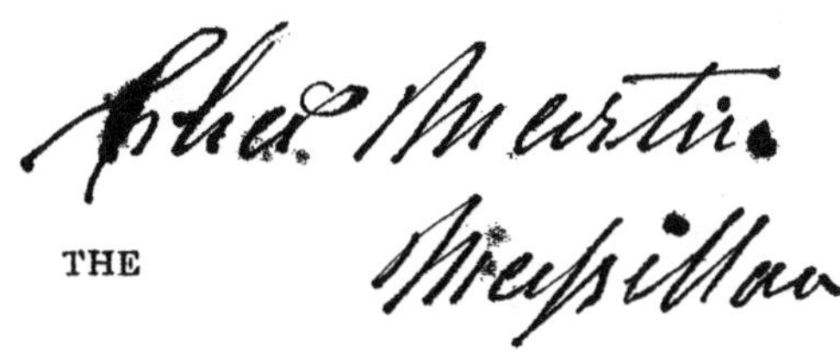

THE

WATER-CURE,

APPLIED TO

EVERY KNOWN DISEASE:

A COMPLETE DEMONSTRATION OF THE ADVANTAGES OF THE HYDROPATHIC SYSTEM OF CURING DISEASES: SHOWING, ALSO, THE FALLACY OF THE MEDICINAL METHOD, AND ITS UTTER INABILITY TO EFFECT A PERMANENT CURE.

WITH AN APPENDIX, CONTAINING A WATER DIET AND RULES FOR BATHING.

BY J. H. RAUSSE,

PRACTITIONER OF WATER-CURE IN MECKLENBURG, GERMANY.

TRANSLATED BY C. H. MEEKER, M. D.,

MEMBER OF THE SCIENTIFIC HYDROPATHIC SOCIETY OF GERMANY

THIRD EDITION, ENLARGED AND IMPROVED.

NEW YORK:

FOWLERS AND WELLS,

CLINTON HALL, 131 NASSAU STREET.

1850.

Miscellen zur Gräfenberger Wasserkur

R. CRAIGHEAD'S POWER PRESS,
112 FULTON STREET.

CONTENTS.

TRANSLATOR'S PREFACE.

I WAS induced to undertake the translation of the present work for several important reasons: first, to employ advantageously several leisure hours of each day, which would otherwise have been entirely wasted or misspent; second, as a means of gaining a more intimate acquaintance with the principles and processes of the hydriatic art, which is to be acquired only by a diligent study of the writings of the most approved authors and practitioners of this new system; third, because it is a most excellent work, containing wonderful and astounding new truths, as every one who reads it must admit; and fourth, because it is written by the most successful and scientific practitioner of hydriatique (the father of the system excepted) in Germany, who spent eight years in studying the various branches of science connected with the water-cure art, though, at first, without the intention of employing his knowledge for the benefit of "suffering humanity," to which he was, however, afterwards induced, from reasons best known to himself. Three years of his study were passed among the Indians of the American wilds in strictly observing nature, and the effects of a life of original simplicity.

In the German language there are also a number of other valuable works, which enjoy a permanent and well-deserved reputation; among others, those of Munde, Krause, and Weiss, are the most prominent. Munde's is a hydrotherapy, though neither original in its conception, nor true to hydriatic principles in its execution; still, in most points, it is an excellent hand-book of water-cure, and stands among the first of all treatises upon the subject in hand, it being a compendious, comprehensive, and highly elaborate work, entering into all the minutiæ of the treatment of the various diseases. Krause's is an excellent hydrotherapy, adhering strictly to the principles and method of treatment pursued by Vincent Priessnitz. The work of Weiss, with whom I also became acquainted while residing at Graefenberg, and had many conversations on the subject of water-cure, has already been laid before the English public, and, consequently, water-cure readers are, to some extent at least, acquainted with its character.

The present work of Rausse, however, is, in its character, conception, and intention, altogether distinct from the above-mentioned; it is not a therapy; it is not to be used as a hand-book to direct the treatment of diseases; it is a true pathology, a doctrine of disease divested of the errors of the old system, retaining only that part of the same which is consistent with true sense and sound reason. It portrays a true picture of the nature of diseases, astonishing us with the sense of the reality that most of the so-called acute diseases are, in truth, a blessing rather than a misfortune, under a correct hydrotherapeutic management; detailing, in particular, and drawing a strict line of antithetical distinction between the medical and hydriatic method of treatment and cure; representing, from all-recognised principles and laws of physiology, the injuriousness of the medical method, and the advantage and lasting benefit accruing from the hydriatic treatment of disease. The American public may judge somewhat of its worth and merits by the fact that, through the influence of the members of the medical profession, the public sale of it was prohibited in the Austrian dominions. Still, it was in the possession of almost every Graefenberg cure-guest, and the work was at first brought to my notice and presented to me by Mr. C. von G., a Tyrolean gentleman of fine talents and excellent disposition, who, I am happy to say, was, before my departure from Graefenberg, quite restored to an excellent state of health; and although not far removed from his third score year of life, and has labored under a complication of the most severe maladies, still avowed that, since his eighteenth year he had never enjoyed better health.

C. H. M.

VINCENT PRIESSNITZ.

THE inclinations and antipathies of instinct are the leading-strings by which Nature directs man and beast on the road to happiness and health. Man is not ordained to independent emancipation from the bonds of Nature; every digression from the voice of Nature is a revolt, an outbreak, and their consequences are misery and affliction. A great part of the human race has burst asunder these bonds, and is consequently broken down and loaded with affliction; it is going the way to destruction.

Salvation is alone possible by a return to Nature, to simplicity —that is virtue. Health is alone possible by abstinence from everything against which the instinct of a man of Nature warns, especially from the poisons which it has pleased man to call Medicines, and from those drinks and potions which the chemical art prepares, and which are enemies to human reason. Cure is alone possible by means of the abundant use of the elements Air and Water!

Such are the thoughts, that lighten, as guiding stars, in all the doings and efforts of Vincent Priessnitz. He does not express them, because he is no friend to many words; he treads the path of his thoughts silent and alone, as the extraordinary among mankind have in all times been wont to do.

He is more than a genius, in the modern sense; he is a wise, i. e. a true man, and, in every respect, a man. Whithersoever he might have turned the eye of his radiant mind, there he would have discovered new truths, and opened new paths of life. Destiny assigned to him the healing of man.

Already a mere youth, he perceived, with searching glance in the structure of the healing art, which centuries have inherited, and on which millions of workmen have labored, a labyrinth full of murderous deceit and error; already, as a mere youth, he had the unshakable courage to form, express, hold firmly, his own opinions in contradiction to the authority of thousands of years, and the belief of millions of men; aye, and to stake his life upon the truths of his opinion. The bold position was won, and with this won, Va-banque! was it decided that, at some future time, the obscure peasant boy of the remote Sudates will blow into air the old title-dressed, order-bedangled art of poisoning.

A youth of eighteen, he cured himself of inflammation of the lungs, and a serious fracture of the ribs, in an incredibly short time, and, by a course which, according to the old healing-art, should have caused his death. So soon as he had obtained these great results, he pursued, with a bold soul eager of discovery, the course he had taken, on an entirely unknown, unnavigated ocean.

The Atlantis, which he was yet to discover, the blessed island of cure, lay afar off, and was veiled and hidden behind the foam of the most fearful breakers. For well may one compare the death-menacing crisis which the water-cure calls up, and through which alone lies the path to the cure of chronic diseases, with the most terrible raging of the waves. Such a crisis, with its burning fever, accompanied, sometimes, with franticness, would have been sufficient to frighten back any common person with terror and trembling from the perplexed path. But Priessnitx remained calm, cool, firm; for to him it was certainty that Nature never deceives, and never leads man into misery, and he was following the dictates of Nature.

Thus he stood undaunted, a second Columbus; he alone

against the barking and ridicule of the old world; thus steered he his bark into the haven of the new.

Now he has the raging and the monsters of the deep behind him; now he stands, the palm-crowned hero, under the palms of the new world, which he has discovered.

Thou that readest this, banish thy smiling until thou hast perused these pages throughout! If then thou still wouldst ridicule, I pray thee desist, go hence to the Sudates, look into the eye of Vincent Priessnitz, behold the tears of joy of those he has saved, and list to the stammering of their thanks.

Go thither to those mountains; there, high above nations' heads, stands the form of that great man, embracing and upholding with one arm the eternal love-dispensing Nature, reaching forth the other to mankind, and offering it restoration to health, happiness, and a new era.

PREFACE TO THE THIRD EDITION.

SINCE writing my first hydriatic pamphlet eight years have elapsed. The enthusiasm for the creation of Vincent Priessnitz which seizes every one who is so fortunate as to find his way into this new spiritual world, directed, at that time, my pen. Enthusiasm is, in its nature, a something ardent and streaming; it moderates either in the course of time, and dissolves into air, or it cools and hardens to an unshakable conviction, whose foundation must rest as well in facts as in reason and science. To such a conviction has my enthusiasm, since the last eight years, cooled and hardened. The facts which I have collected in these eight years, indeed, first, in a great number of private cures, afterwards in a water-cure establishment, founded and directed by myself, all these consonant facts have furnished me the proof that the water-cure method is the only right one, and that the theory of the water-cure art, and the doctrine of disease, detected and brought forward by me, is, in all points of chief moment, truth. I must confess that, in affairs of secondary importance, I have sometimes erred; especially in the first editions of my works, there are errors present in regard to the practical detail-application of water. The practical errors of the first editions consist wholly in recommendation of an excessive use of water and too cold degree of temperature. Without here investigating the causes whence the excesses in the water-cure originate, I may herewith excuse my former faults, on the ground that originally Vincent Priessnitz himself had fallen into many excesses, and that every patient, as soon as he wins full confidence in the hydriatique, carries the use of water, at first, to excess. I have never yet witnessed an exception to this rule, for which reason I warn every new cure-guest on entering my establishment against overstepping my directions; while at the same time, I feel assured, and apprise the patient of my conviction, that he will still surpass the prescribed limits. Farthermore, I have formerly represented, in exaggerated terms, the beneficial effects of the water-cure art in chronic diseases, not intentionally, however, but from the error into which enthusiasm so easily leads. My eight years' experience has convinced me that the effects of medicinal poisonings cannot, in all chronic diseases, be *completely* removed by the water-cure, because these poisonings often enough occasion such organic changes or ravages that they then still partially continue when the medicinal poisons are driven out of the body through the agency of water.

But, on the other hand, I have, by the experience and the most diligent research of these eight years, been confirmed in the conviction and the knowledge that, hard as I have in the first editions of my writings judged of the medical method of cure, still I have not done it injustice, and in that case, have been guilty of no exaggeration. I have been convinced that, in all diseases, the medicinal means of cure can produce only increased misfortunes of disease, even if in acute diseases they are of *apparent* good; I have been farther convinced, that there is no disease and no state of disease in which the greatest possible assistance and benefit cannot be afforded by the water-cure.

This book contains the physiological and pathological demonstration, why the medical method of cure must always be injurious. It contains at the same time, and first of all, the outline of a new doctrine of disease, which is deduced as much from the results of the new method of cure as from recognised physiological rules and fundamental principles. It is farther proved in this work that the pathology and therapy of the physicians stand in contradiction with the physiology which these physicians recognise and teach from their professorial chairs, and that the doctrine of disease first discovered by me, and brought forward in this book, contains nothing which is not a consequence fairly drawn from well-known physiological rules. In accordance with the foregoing, it need scarcely be observed, that this book is no therapy, and that no one may expect, with the assistance of this alone, to conduct water-cures. I insert here a warning against water-cures on one's own responsibility, unaltered from the preface of the second edition of this work, for this reason, that no one may attribute this warning to selfish motives, because at that time, and for three years after, I neither had a water-cure establishment nor the intention to undertake the practice of hydriatique as a vocation.

On page vii of the second edition it reads thus:—

"Many persons, as soon as they have gained confidence in the water-cure, commence immediately to treat themselves, on their own responsibility, presuming that no especial requirements and experience are necessary to this method of cure. That is a dangerous error, which has already done much injury, as well to such persons as to the water-cure. Even under the direction of a *distant* water-physician, the consequence of the treatment is, at the best, doubtful, since misconceptions of many kinds cannot but arise. If Priessnitz knew how strangely wrong many of his correspondence-patients understood and pursued his directions, how inclined most are, in the alarm of a crisis, to have recourse to a mediciner, and how much less judgment people in general possess, than he attributes to them, I believe that Priessnitz would wish to renounce all correspondence-practice. Where then any one, through his own errors, grows worse instead of better, then he accuses the water, while he should only lament his own want of judgment. Most mediciners hail such unfortunate events as real blessed turns of fortune, which they employ in order, with loud voice, to warn their unfortunate patients against the water-cure, and to retain them in the medical.

"Such mishaps can only be obviated by a comprehensive and universally serviceable hand-book of hydrotherapeutics. Munde has already supplied one, serviceable in some respects and particulars, namely, serviceable for those who have also visited a hydropathic establishment, and then only in certain states of disease. But his book lacks much of being a comprehensive and generally serviceable guide for all persons in all diseases. Mr. Munde lacks all capability to the literary improvement of the hydriatique; he lacks the talent to bring within the scope of the understanding the principles of hydrotherapeutics, ofttimes practised by Priessnitz in the never-erring instinct of an intuitive geniality, and adapt the peculiar good of the genius to the general good of all men. It does not belong in this place to prove that also all future attempts at therapeutic hand-books must necessarily prove abortive, even in their birth, if they are constructed upon the hitherto customary principles (which Munde has also followed); still less can the new therapeutic principles be unfolded, which, moreover, are nothing else than consequences deducible from the pathological fundamental truths given in this work."

A cursory comparison of this third edition with the second will convince the reader that this book has undergone an entire change, partly through erasure, partly through retouching, and partly through addition of considerable extra matter.

When in this work I speak of physicians in general, of the incorrigibility of their professional errors and prejudices, of the conceitedness and arrogance of the sect, of their indifference to truth, of their tender sensibility for the interests of their purse, I would not have it understood that, by this general censure, I exclude, or dispute, in any wise, numerous honorable exceptions. Under all classes the common souls compose the majority: under all classes are to be found individual noble men, to whom truth is dearer than private emolument. Already many truth loving physicians have altered materially in their practice, and these changes will, in future, occur yet more frequently. But the "servum pecus" of common receipt-blotters will persevere in their old habits, either from error or self-interest, so long as the same can be made a lucrative business.

J. H. R.

Stuer, December, 1845.

A.

THE POWER OF APPROPRIATION

AND

SECRETION IN GENERAL.

The power of appropriation, of assimilation of foreign substance into one's self; into bodily I, is the fundamental principle upon which Nature has built her system.

This propensity and this power is not only in all organic bodies, the predominant, but also in the elementary bodies.*

In the beginning the globe was a bleak rock, upon which the air and water exercised their power of appropriation.

Appropriation can be effected only by decomposition. In order to appropriate, the air and water decomposed the

* The words "elementary bodies, elements," are here employed in the old popular sense, in which they signify, "Air, Earth, Fire, Water;" consequently not in the chemical sense, in which they denote "chemically indecomposable substances" in contra-distinction to the compound.

earth's crust, thus originated the dissolved surface capable of producing and maintaining organic beings.

Since these beings—beasts and plants, are intended to live in a world wherein the elements constantly exercise on all matter their power of decomposition and appropriation: therefore from the beginning the same power must have developed itself as primary and fundamental power in the organic beings for a defence against the elements.

Instances of the appropriating propensity of the elements among one another are: The air decomposes the water in vapors, in order to appropriate to itself its gases. Water again absorbs from the air oxygen gas. Fire devours the oxygen gas of the air again; it frees water into its two elements, viz. hydrogen and oxygen gas, and thus by burning these gases it transforms water into fire. The air absorbs many gases, which fire sets free. The air draws gases from the earth, the earth draws oxygen gas from the air. Thus the elements stand in constant strife with each other; each endeavors to decompose the other, and wholly appropriate its elements to itself.

Instances of the strife of assimilation between the elements and organisms are: The organic bodies draw in from the air oxygen gas through the respiratory process, which dwells also in all plants; the organic bodies (plants) draw through the absorption of the roots or (beasts) by the consumption of plants, into their own substance all that, which the earth's soil offers them capable of assimilation. Vice versâ fire decomposes and assimilates all organisms and their products; water and air endeavor to effect the same on the organic beings, which, while they are alive, is accomplished only in part by appropriation of the evaporations, after their death, however, entirely. The earth exercises upon living organisms this power only conditionally and partially, namely, when their residence is in the earth, as for instance many beasts live there, and all the roots of plants. On man the earth does not generally exercise decomposition until life has become extinct (unless on those who use the dirt baths of Dr. Graham, which Lichtenberg classes among the materia medica, because they sometimes perhaps do no injury).

The earth, however, exercises somewhat of this power also upon those living human beings, who in the savage state live in caves of the earth, or sleep on the bare ground. To these belong especially most tribes in New Holland.

This power is the co-operating cause, which, even when there is no taking of cold in the question, produces a commotion in the body after sleep on the bare ground, and when this is treated in the medical manner, degenerates into a real disease. Therefore people usually say, the exhalations from the earth are unwholesome ; but they are so only for the effeminate, and those weaned from Nature.

Instances of the strife of assimilation among the organisms themselves are : Beasts devour each other and plants ; that is, they appropriate to themselves, with the help of the stomach, so much of their substance as can be assimilated by them. Plants, on the other hand, transform many parts of dead beasts and plants (dung) into their own substance.

Besides this power of assimilation and the power of reaction against foreign attempts at decomposition, it is still requisite for each being, element, and organism, to be exposed to the influence of foreign appropriative power.

That is the fundamental principle of the doctrine of healing.

Instances of this principle : Water becomes thick and putrid if withdrawn from the decomposing power of agitated air ; the air loses its oxygenous principle and becomes mephitic if it find no water and no vegetables with which to exercise reciprocally its decomposing and assimilating power. Beasts and plants sicken and die when their surface is so covered that neither air nor water can exercise their decomposing power upon it.

When nutriment is withdrawn from an organic being, i. e. the opportunity to appropriate to itself foreign matter, then death follows from a failure of the supply to the juices of the body ; if, on the contrary, this being is withdrawn from the influence of foreign decomposing power, disease follows from the coagulation and corruption of the juices from want of the removal of refuse humors by the power of foreign appropriation.

B.

THE POWER OF APPROPRIATION

AND SECRETION OF THE

ANIMAL ORGANISMS IN PARTICULAR.

THE condition of vitality in general has not as yet been thoroughly investigated by any one, still less its classification in species, varieties, and individual cases.

Individual powers and processes of vitality have been explored, and we are accustomed to call the systematically arranged doctrine of these processes the physiology of plants and beasts.

Under the as yet known laws of physiology (we are here concerned only with the animal physiology) the law of appropriation and secretion is one of the most general importance, and in the relation it bears to the healing art, decidedly the chief. The renovation of the substance in animal bodies is the necessary consequence of this law, which renovation extends itself to the innermost and most solid parts, viz. the bones, i. e. all parts of the animal bodies receive into themselves daily foreign matter, and incorporate it into a part of themselves (they make it similar to themselves, hence the words assimilate, assimilation); in like manner these bodies excrete somewhat of their own substance, and thus renew by degrees their whole substance.

Learned naturalists have produced learned proofs for the existence of the above mentioned laws, which, however, are very superfluous for the true thinker, since the one untaught perspicuous fact that no animal organism can survive without nutriment (i. e. sustain itself spontaneously in its separate individuality from the external world), furnishes to the thinker the proof of the law of assimilation and secretion, and consequently of the law of the change of matter in the animal bodies.

For if none of the aliment of animals were transformed into their own essential substance, then this whole aliment would again pass off without being used, and would be quite superfluous; consequently animals would be spared the numerous sufferings arising from want of nourishment, and from the endeavors to procure it. This is, however, impossible, because there is no absurd law to be found in Nature. If, however, much of the nutriment is incorporated by the animal bodies into their essence, then on the other hand much of this must be again secreted, because otherwise the body would constantly increase in weight just as much as the weight of the food which is assimilated. (The secretions, however, are to be divided into such as consist in unemployed, unserviceable aliment, and in such as consist in refuse matter of the organism itself.)

I must, however, because I live in a more learned than thinking age, bring forward also some learned detail proofs of the transformation of matter in animals. Readers who do not love learnedness, may omit the same.

1st. In anatomical examinations we notice plainly a certain alteration in young and old bodies, viz. increase of the earthy and fibrous matter, and decrease of the glutinous and serous. This alteration does not arise from disease as an exception to the general rule, but normally, and always from old age.

2d. The bones of beasts become red, when they are fed with madder.

3d. The roots of the milk teeth disappear.

4th. The bones in advanced age decrease in circumference and weight.

5th. Cartilage changes into bony matter, and thus cartilaginous substance disappears.

It is not so difficult to show in what manner solid matter is transformed into liquid in the animal bodies, as is the explanation of the manner of forming solid from fluid matters; the latter comes more conspicuously to notice, when the bones, in the growing season of life, are increasing, which are undoubtedly formed directly and indirectly from the blood.

The transformation of the liquid into solid is thus: on the extremities of the arteries, there where they deposit serum on the fibres, the blood loses oxygen gas, which transforms the liquid serum into solid matter.

The change of the solid into liquid takes place in the following manner: the absorbent vessels (vasa absorbentia) or lymphatic veins (venae lymphaticae serosae) soften solid substances by moisture and absorption, they conduct absorbed liquids out of the limbs into the body, and empty themselves through the main trunk of the veins in the back part of the breast into the left collar bone vein (vena subclavia sinistra) and in the right jugular vein (vena jugularis dextra); solid parts having in this manner been made liquid, and conducted into the above-mentioned veins, the discharge of the liquid takes place through the organ of the skin, further by the aid of the glands from the hollows of the eyes, of the ears, and of the nose, further also partially through the bladder and rectum.

The processes, also, whereby on the one hand the formation, maintenance, and increase of the bones, whereby on the other hand the removal of refuse matter from the body is carried on, have already been followed out in detail by learned physiologists, and exposed to view.

Many kinds of experiments, which have been confirmed also by Troja's method, have shown that the formation, growth, and sustenance of the bones proceed from the external periosteum, the absorption, however, from the internal or skin of the marrow.

The following facts relate thereto:

1. When the skin of the marrow has been destroyed, the bone dies, whereupon a new skin to the marrow, and a new piece of bone grows instead.

2. This latter forms itself between the new skin of the marrow and the periosteum.

3. These two skins form together only one very thick skin, divisible into laminae.

4. The new skin of the marrow separates by degrees from the periosteum by the interposition of the new bone.

5. The texture of the skin of the marrow, which is at first very thick and close, becomes gradually more tender, fills with juices, and at last becomes precisely similar to the former skin.

6. The inner surface of the new skin of the marrow, which exhibits alternately elevations and depressions, dis-

solves and destroys the old bone, and absorbs it completely. When the medullary skin of the end of an amputated bone is separated with a stilet, the untouched skin of the leg begins to swell; there arises on the outward surface of the bone a layer of cartilage, which originates in the skin of the leg, with which it is intimately connected, and from which the new springs.

The exchange of matter in the organic beings, as well as in the elements, is an evident truth, which to my knowledge has not been disputed by any naturalist since the discovery of that law. This exchange in the organic beings is only possible through liquefaction of the solid matter, and on the other hand through consolidation of the liquid matter. These unceasingly successive transformations can only be effected by means of oxygen and hydrogen, since the oxygen hardens the liquid, and the hydrogen softens the solid matter, as has been proved by many concurring investigations and experiments, among others by the discovery first made by Dr. Curssel, in Petersburg, that flesh on the oxygen pole of the galvanic chain became hard, and on the hydrogen pole became soft. Curssel has proved, on many other substances, the solvent power of the hydrogen pole, and the desiccating hardening power of the oxygen pole.

From the foregoing principles we make the following deductions:

1. Water, as is known, consists of hydrogen and oxygen; 2. and moreover, that these constituent parts of water effect the transformation and exchange of matter in the organic beings; 3. to this we add, in conclusion, that the undisturbed and normal exchange of matter in the body is the fundamental condition of the life and health of or-

ganic beings. From these three data taken together, we draw the conclusion, that water is the chief material of health and cure for the organic body, and consequently that the Water-cure method is the correct method, and deeply and eternally founded in nature.

Whoever is not yet enabled by the foregoing to discover the small connecting members between the deductions brought forward, will find them farther on, and also the detail proofs of the above made inferences.

C.

WHAT IS INSTINCT?

The law of assimilation and secretion, which with certainty governs the terrestrial creation, and with probability the whole universe, produces manifold collisions and conflicts among the various beings respecting the substance to be assimilated. Also the existence of beasts of prey in the animal kingdom is a consequence of this law. The philosophical consequences of this law are very important, especially for the vindication of optimism; however, they belong not in this book.

To reconcile the collisions and conflicts which take place in procuring matter for assimilation with the continuance and propagation of the various races, was without doubt one of the most important problems for the creative principle, which has been solved with the most eminent and admirable wisdom.

Numberless dangers on all sides and from all the kingdoms of nature threaten young inexperienced animals (we wish to turn our attention to the animal kingdom only). How were it possible to afford them a protection against those dangers, since experience and knowledge are not innate? The assertion that the parents take care of their young till they become of full age, is, from many reasons, entirely untenable. The first reason is the falsity of the thing asserted. Never, in a state of nature, do the parents remain with their young till their full growth, and the great mass of animals never get sight of their parents, viz. fishes, insects, and amphibious animals do not, which come from eggs, the hatching of which is committed to the sun.

What a multitude of dangers is there for animals in the vegetable kingdom alone from the presence of poisons! What a still greater multitude in the animal kingdom from the assimilating enemies, generally called beasts of prey! How was it possible, then, in a creation, wherein the law of assimilation rules supreme, to insure the continuation of the various races? It was possible through the Instinct alone, which nature has bestowed on individuals.

WHAT IS INSTINCT?

That is the question which the learned of all times have variously answered, and these extremely learned explanations have for the most part ended in a literal sense without sense.

WHAT IS INSTINCT?

Ah, that is so simple, easy a question, that any uncorrupted plain human understanding can give but one and the same answer. *Instinct is the purely sensual faculty of all animal creatures, to distinguish by perception of the agreeable and disagreeable, what is conducive to health and life, from what is prejudicial, to seek the former and shun the latter.*

Not man alone possesses this sensual faculty in common with the beasts, but every animal organism on every star of the universe must of absolute necessity be endowed with it, if the law of assimilation and excretion reigns there as on the earth.

Why whimpers the new born babe after the mother's breast? He has a craving for it, because it is necessary to his existence,—that is already instinct. Why are the smell and taste of all poisons disgusting and painful to the man of nature? In order to withhold him from partaking of things destructive to his health—through instinct. Even in this age of refinement the guide-posts of instinct are possessed in part by all. There is no poison, which, when unmixed with other things agreeable to the taste, will not cause disgust and shuddering to every palate, and excite vomiting. However, when a little poison is combined with a great deal of wholesome matter, as alcohol in wine, with delicious fruits and sugar delicacies, then the palate can be deceived, and thus gradually be corrupted. The natural palate, when moistened by any intoxicating liquor, becomes alarmed, as all seamen and discoverers unanimously inform us, that every savage spits out the first draught of anything intoxicating, or perhaps swallows it with averseness and feelings of disgust. This is related by the South sea voyagers, Cook, Bougainville, Dumont d'Urville, and all others. Of course, however, the first warning of instinct is soon overcome by intoxicating stimulants, the instinct-nerves are soon poisoned, and the toper is made. The idolatrous respect of the savages for the gods of thunder, whom they try to imitate in everything, is to blame, that they all after a longer association with Europeans overcome that warning and learn to drink. Farther, man and every beast, that is liable to be poisoned by the bite of snakes, feel, through instinct, without the help of experience or any warning, a shuddering, fear, and deadly enmity at the sight of all serpents, and either flee from them, or take the precaution to kill them. On the contrary, the hog, which is in no wise injured by their bite, exhibits no symptoms of fear, but searches for snakes as for caterpillars or acorns, and devours them; the same is the case with the stork and crane. The proud king lion flees from the scorpion: in his cage it makes him tremble and cringe with fear into the farthest corner; the colossal elephant exhibits the same symptoms towards that minute insect, which creeps into its trunk, and thence into its brain, and thus causes its death.

All the warnings of instinct are entirely innate and need not the cultivation of experience, which constitutes wisdom. Instinct confines itself to the absolute questions of life, and is absolutely infallible. Wisdom presumes to see and explore farther, and is very deceptive.

As the instinct is absolutely infallible, just so absolutely necessary is it to the continuation of our race; every animal tribe, that corrupts the instinct, and destroys it in itself must come to ruin, and it requires not much acuteness to perceive, that the human race is travelling or decaying on towards death; salvation is alone possible, if it regains instinct and nature, which is still possible.

At all events the human species has many thousand years to run on before its total extinction, although every species of beast would have become extinct; for through the whole chain of animal organisms this law prevails, that the more perfect a species is in regard to its physical constitution, it has in the same degree a limited instinct and extended capacity for wisdom, and of the mental and arbitrary functions; thus in the latter capacity it finds a sort of surrogate, but one very deceptive for a deadened instinct. In the most intimate harmony and connexion with that first law stands the second, that the senses are less reliable for the instinct in the same order in which they are nobler, more spiritual and perceptive, thus in the following order: feeling and taste about equal, then smell, hearing, and sight. Of this we mention an explanatory instance. The young hare can sometimes be ensnared by the fox, when the latter dances about him, imitating the pranks of a young hare, so long as the hare is aided by no other sense than that of sight; but as soon as he hears the voice of the beast of prey, or gets scent thereof, he is undeceived, and makes his escape, if it be not already too late. On that account the fox always endeavors to remain under cover of the wind—that is already wisdom, of which the higher orders of beasts are decidedly capable, and oftentimes to an astonishing degree; however, more on this point belongs not here.

With these and similar fundamental features in the nature of the animal organisms the learned naturalists have but little troubled themselves; with most of these gentlemen Nature is nothing else than a naturalist's cabinet with beetles and herbaria, and they are content with classifying salamanders, toads, lice, and caterpillars; alas let those vermin rest in peace until you have explored human nature!

From the foregoing explanation concerning the nature

of instinct, and from the law of assimilation and secretion taken together, it follows, that the means to the continuation of life and health are revealed to animals by their physical impulses.

In like manner, when sickness occurs, the means of cure must be indicated by the same instinct. This second position follows as a consequence of the first; it is however likewise a postulate of reason, that the capability of choosing correctly by *infallible means* those things necessary to their well-being should be bestowed upon animals of a reasonable creation. This capability must in like disposition be distributed through all grades of the animal creation, and must therefore consist in a revelation of the sensual feeling, and not in a function of the mental energy, or in a result of experience, still less of true science, but least of all in the results of a half silly science like the medical.

It follows from the foregoing, that animals falling sick have a sensual desire for the means of cure proper for them, and realize a sensual pleasure in the use of the same. In all primary diseases (concerning this see farther on) this is really the case, inasmuch as every man (beasts still more) has a strong desire for the cooling stimulus and refreshment of water; and in the use of the same experiences a sensual gratification and comfort. (Farther on I will show, how the instinct of man becomes partially corrupted by poisoning, and how in the secondary diseases it is never quite infallible, and is sometimes directly false.)

It follows finally from those arrangements of nature, of which we are speaking, that such pretended means of cure, against which the instinct of the patient and of every healthy man feels averseness and disgust, must be wrong and injurious. Herein then is contained the second proof of the falsity and perniciousness of the medicinal method of cure, because the instinct is infallible.

The sum of all practical wisdom is the rule, obediently to acquiesce in the arrangements and follow the voice of nature—for it is the voice of God; the sum of all theoretical wisdom is the knowledge of the reasons, why all the contrivances of nature must so be, as they are. The sum of all folly, and the fountain of all corruption, is the rebellion against the regulations of nature, and the endeavor to find fault with and tutor them.

In this unfortunate direction of folly, there has been no human or scientific error in so high a degree fatal and silly as the medicinal method of cure.

D.

SIGNIFICATION OF THE TERMS

"HEALTH AND DISEASE."

Before I commence defining the terms health and disease, I must observe, that there are in reality no species or varieties definitely marked off from one another; that the individuals of every species and variety have dissimilarities among themselves; that the transitions, from one species to the other are so imperceptible, that with certain individuals and concrete cases it cannot be determined with certainty to which species they belong. This is particularly the case with the different diseases, and even the line of demarcation between health and disease is in cases of reality frequently very wavering. In a word, the denominations of species, &c., are not borrowed from reality, and thence delivered over to human ingenuity, but vice versâ, have originated in the human mind, and from there been transferred to the reality, because the former cannot operate without them. Whoever wishes to read more upon this subject, I refer to the introduction to my "Guide to the Practice of the Water Cure System," soon to appear, where I was obliged to enter into the depth of this thema.

The disposition of vitality in the organic beings in regard to duration of time may be called double; namely, the vital energy may be of such a kind that it wears itself out gradually by the labor of appropriation and excretion, by the strife with the appropriative power of the external world, and finally perishes. Organic beings, that are endowed with such vitality, can effectuate the continuance of their species only through propagation and births. Of this kind are the organic beings of our planet.

We may suppose that, upon other bodies of the universe and, viz. upon the self-existent stars, which we call fixed stars, there may exist beings materially organic of a higher nature, whose vital energy does not wear out, and consequently does not perish. With such beings propagation may be dispensed with, because the race continues on without it, and it must be dispensed with, because the propensity thereto is incompatible with an exalted nature, and because probably no constantly even and eternally enduring vitality of individuals is compatible with the capability and exercise of the propagation of the race.

Among the physiological and psychological laws known to us, there is none that sets a contradiction between the notions of immortality and materiality of any being.

In accordance with these two essentially different kinds of vitality, the notions of absolute health are just as essentially different. The idea of the absolute health of a being not having necessarily self-consuming vitality, coincides with the everlasting life of that being. The idea of the absolute health of a being possessing necessarily self-extinguishing vitality, is quite a different one. In the latter case, not only the death, but also the earlier or later occurrence thereof, give no certain principle whereby to determine the idea of absolute health. This conception is chiefly determined by two indications, viz. first, in freedom from pain during the whole course of life ; and second, in the harmony of the functions, and the *proportionate* diminution of the functions in entering upon that age which lies between the noonday of life and death. Finally, the following condition (which has already been indirectly inferred in the two first-mentioned indications) is included in the conception of the absolute health of a being with vitality necessarily self-consuming, viz. that death in good old age must occur without pain. Such a death deserves the name of a normal and healthy death, while on the contrary, every death connected with a struggle is a death by disease. It is undeniable, that such absolute health occurs but in very few instances with the animal creations of our planet, even when in a state of nature, if we include in the term sickness all the numberless and petty injuries inflicted through external violence. When this is not the case, then absolute health occurs much oftener, although by no means always, because, upon our planet, animals even in a state of health are subject to epidemic diseases, which probably have their originating cause in periodical corruption of the elements ; of this see farther on.

E.

DIVISION OF THE

CAUSES OF DISEASE INTO CLASSES.

If we take the term disease in the broadest signification of the word, then the causes of disease resolve themselves into four several classes:

Namely, first, In injuries inflicted by external objects.

Second, In destroying the balance of the functions through over-exercise of individual organs; for example, of the organ of sight, of thought, of procreation.

Third, In destroying the same balance through injuries and fearful affections of the mind.

Fourth, In the burdening of the animal organism with foreign matters internally (matters of disease). The foreign matters of disease fall into two several principal classes, viz. first, into actual matter, which is foreign to the organism, but is not in a normal manner promptly excreted, from want of some of the conditions of excretion, of which farther on much will be said. Second, Into such matters of the external world as are introduced into the body through the organs of the skin or stomach, and which from beginning to end are incapable of being assimilated (poisons).

The causes of diseases given under 2 and 3 are extremely seldom present by themselves, they are almost always more or less combined with the matters of disease given under division 4. In the very seldom cases in which they may be present alone, to cure them it is necessary only to remove the *causes* of the disease. We do not occupy ourselves at all in this work with the second and third causes of disease as existing of themselves alone, and on this account, because in reality they extremely seldom appear, and secondly, because for them there is no positive, but only a negative method of cure, and thirdly, because all signs of reaction fail them. (See farther on.)

A fifth class of causes of bodily suffering, which arise from insufficient nourishment and over-driven exertion of the whole body, is accordingly excluded from this work, because these noxious influences bring suffering only upon the organic body, but no disease, if they, to wit, are by themselves alone and not connected with any grand cause of disease in the body.

The class of disease given under division 4, will first be treated of in this work as by far the most important, and the first class of disease will then follow as appendant.

F.

CLASSIFICATION

OF DISEASES THEMSELVES;

DIFFERENT MODES OF CLASSIFICATION.

In the Introduction to the "Guide to the Practice of the Water-Cure Art," I have in detailed manner shown, that in reality there are no classes among diseases, but only cases or individual instances of disease, no two of which are precisely alike, many of which, however, are similar, and according to this similarity constitute groups natural, but not strictly separate from one another. These groups, which are natural and run into each other, have by the human mind been arranged into classes, or in species and varieties, because it cannot work without specific ideas. have in the above-mentioned introduction shown, that no doctrine of disease is possible without classification of the diseases in species and varieties according to their several natures, and that on the other hand no doctrine of cure with such a classification according to the nature of the *diseases* can have a practical usefulness.

The arrangement of diseases in species and varieties

may be based on very various and different signatures of classification (a signature of classification is a mark which gives the rule wherewith to direct the arrangement into classes or into species and varieties). The duration of the diseases, for instance, may be set up as the rule to direct the arrangement, the nature of the matter of disease, or the physiological system of the body, in which the disease has its seat (the glandular system, the muscular system, or osseous system), or the anatomical part of the body which is affected (whether head, breast, or abdomen), may be taken to direct the rule of classification, &c.

If the division of diseases into classes and sorts actually existed, then it would be possible to discover some one signature of classification, in conformity with which the construction of the whole doctrine of disease could be strictly and definitely carried out. The fact, that pathologists have not succeeded in the arrangement of diseases in strict truth and consecution according to one single signature of classification, consequently explains itself very naturally from this circumstance, that the division of the divers sorts of diseases into classes does not at all exist in the *reality*. The labors of many pathologists in endeavoring to arrange and fabricate the system of pathology in conformity with one signature of classification testify to the want of sense of these learned persons, and to their misapprehension of the truth, that in the *reality* there are no classes of diseases. Such systems bear in themselves the double stamp of being both untrue and forced. Whoever has perceived that the classification of diseases is an untruth in the reality, but for the operations and researches of the human mind an indispensable crutch, such an one gives himself not a moment's trouble to bring the whole territory of pathology under one single signature of classification, and he is guided in the choice of his different signatures, not by the endeavor to attain to philosophical strictness, but simply in consideration of making himself intelligible to readers.

In this work we divide diseases into four principal classes, namely:

1. In healing diseases.
2. In destroying diseases.
3. In infectious and epidemic diseases.
4. In external or surgical diseases.

The healing diseases coincide for the most part, but not altogether, with those diseases which physicians call "acute," and the destroying diseases with those which are usually comprehended under the name "chronic diseases."

Observation: Acute diseases are, according to the definition of the physicians, "such as do not last over four weeks, generally accompanied by fever, and confine to the bed. Chronic diseases, on the other hand, are such as generally do not confine to the bed, whose duration is over four weeks, and are commonly unattended with fever."

The unserviceableness of this mode of classification, taken from the mere surface, comes plainly into view when we consider that one minute's difference in the duration of the disease can make no essential point of distinction. Generally speaking, the duration of diseases is a mode of classifying which characterizes the nature of diseases little or not at all, and consequently does not enter into the depth of pathology. When, in the former editions of my hydriatic writings, I received as normal the division of diseases into acute and chronic, it was only because I made use of these two words in a quite new signification. Namely, in the divisions made first by myself of diseases into healing and destroying diseases, I used the word "acute" for the first class, and the word "chronic" for the second. Such an altered manner of employing old medical terms, however, occasions misunderstandings, and on this account I have exchanged these old names for such new ones as are more suited to my new system of pathology, and subject to no misunderstanding. If in this third edition, also, the words "acute" and "chronic" should still remain in some places, I pray you attribute it to the press for time under which I must undertake the revision of this edition. Instead thereof the words "primary" and "secondary" disease will be found—"primary" answering to the healing diseases, "secondary" to the class of destroying diseases. The reasons which determined me in the use of these terms will be found farther on.

G.

THE SYMPTOMS OF DISEASES,

AND

CLASSIFICATION OF THE SAME.

In the following section H. the materiality of the causes of disease will be treated of, and proved. Here the position that the causes, if not of all, yet of nearly all, diseases are foreign matters in the diseased organism, must be anticipated and premised previous to its proof. Accordingly, then, disease itself consists in the burdening of the organism internally with foreign matters, particularly with acrid, corrosive, putrid, universally with matters more or less poisonous.

Those expressions of disease manifesting themselves externally to the perception, we call signs or symptoms of the disease, well aware that we employ these words in a signification widely differing from the medical terminology, which, indeed, cannot be otherwise, since here we have to do with a doctrine of disease entirely new. Disease comes to the perception of the patient himself through his general feeling always, and through the senses of sight, of smell, of hearing, and of touch sometimes,—to the observing physician, through one or more of the last named senses.

The symptoms of disease resolve themselves, according to their inmost nature, into symptoms of the organic struggle against the matter of disease in the body, and the destructive effects of this matter upon the organic body. The first symptoms we will call symptoms of reaction, because they arise from the reaction of the system against the matters of disease, i. e. disease-causing matters. Accordingly the symptoms of reaction arise from the endeavor of the organism to heal itself, to rid itself of its disturbing matter, and might therefore be called healing symptoms, if we did not need this word for a subdivision of the symptoms of reaction, namely, for those symptoms of reaction to which belong the signs of the *success* of the reaction, i. e. of the victory of the organism over its disease-causing matters. The symptoms of reaction include also those symptoms which are as yet only endeavors of the organism to rid itself of the disease, even if those endeavors fail.

In all internal diseases not produced by external injuries, every severe pain, and every severe (acute) inflammation is decidedly a symptom of reaction.

The second class of symptoms of disease consists in the destructive effects of the matters of disease upon the organism, and these symptoms we will call destroying symptoms or "passive symptoms of disease." The term, "active symptoms of disease" would be perfectly expressive for the symptoms of reaction.

The passive or the destroying symptoms consist in organic destructions through ulceration, fistula and cancer-sores, in organic transformations, ossification, enlargements, contractions, accumulations of diseased fluid humors (dropsy); farther, in cramps of the most various kinds, &c., &c.

The symptoms of reaction in their perfection, totality, and greatest strength, are only to be found in the primary or healing diseases. They aim at the radical cure, the complete expulsion of all disturbing matters of disease. There are, however, in the chronic diseases also imperfect symptoms of reaction, i. e. signs of the contra-working of the organism against the extension of the matters of disease, a struggle not for radical cure of the disease, but for preservation of the status quo, for suppression of the disease as long as possible. We need, therefore, a distinction between the symptoms of reaction in primary (acute) and secondary (chronic) diseases, and we will call the first absolute or total signs of reaction, the second, relative or partial signs of reaction.

Since now, in the foregoing, we have erected the framework of our mode of classification and terminology, we can, in what follows, enter upon the matter itself, because we now understand each other. I am well aware how tedious the foregoing must have been to the reader, but it could not be otherwise; classification and terminology are always necessary, and both must be created anew, if one wishes to bring into the world a group of new truths.

H.

PROOFS FOR THE MATERIALITY OF THE

CAUSES OF DISEASE

OR FOR THE

EXISTENCE OF MATTERS OF DISEASE.

My whole doctrine of disease rests upon two fundamental positions, namely:

1. Upon the position that foreign material substances are the causes of perfect diseases (of this see directly below), and 2, upon the position that all diseases resolve themselves into the essentially different classes of healing and destroying diseases.

In the special pathology, farther on, will be found the detail proof of these two positions in relation to each individual sort of disease. Here we must first bring forward the proofs for both of these positions in general, which philosophy, physiology, and daily experience, i. e. the perception of the senses, furnish, so that hereafter in the special pathology, in the detailed statement of the sickening and healing processes, the basis of the whole conclusion of this work may be ready at hand, without which basis, the reader might think the later conclusions float in the air, and are petitiones principii.

In this section, H., we shall take up only the first of my two fundamental positions, and consider the second afterwards in course.

When I say that material foreign substances are the causes of all perfect diseases, I understand by perfect diseases those that are accompanied with symptoms of reaction, or have been preceded by such symptoms. To the symptoms of reaction belong particularly all kinds of pain and all kinds of inflammation. We perceive from this definition the extreme rarity of imperfect diseases not combined with matters of disease. It is an extremely rare circumstance that a person gets diseased without ever in his life having had a pain or inflammation, and that his disease likewise arises and runs its course without both of these symptoms. We might name the imperfect or reactionless diseases, also dynamic, and the perfect ones, chemical (as regards their causes), however, in the argument concerning the existence of disease-causing matter I could not choose these names if I wished to be free from all objections.

In a later edition of this work I will devote an appropriate part to the imperfect diseases; now time fails me for that purpose, which also compels me to leave unconsidered those abnormities which originate in the natural false structure of the body and its organs, and which are likewise destitute of symptoms of reaction, and moreover do not admit of cure.

Accordingly, when in this edition we speak of diseases, only those attended with signs of reaction, or the perfect diseases, are intended.

Two proofs of the most different kind can be adduced in confirmation of the existence of the materiality of all perfect diseases, namely, a philosophical proof upon the principles of Deism and optimism, and a proof from facts drawn from the perception of the senses.

A.

THE PHILOSOPHICAL PROOF.

If the causes of diseases are material, man can avoid them, because these disease-producing matters can only get into his body in a manner which comes to the knowledge of his senses, and which excites aversion, disgust, and even horror in every healthy and uncorrupted person, since instinct revolts against it.

This feeling speaks plainly against all sharp and poisonous substances, when they are introduced into the body either through the swallow or through the skin.

If then the causes of disease are material, and are substances more or less poisonous within the body, man has in his own self a warner and safeguard against disease—and it must be so if we do not admit that man in his very creation is a marred and imperfect being, which would condition therefore an imperfect total creation. Only a fool can believe this; the wise man finds the older he grows, the deeper he penetrates into the spirit of the creation, the more justifications of the apparent improprieties in the creation, and the more grounds for the acceptation of a most exalted wisdom. The evils which come upon the human race are not the consequences of perverted creation, but of perverted application of our own powers and our own freedom. Thus it must be; every being must bear in its own self the capability of being happy.

In the acceptation of the so-called dynamic theories, which, since Haller, have been the ruling in medicine, the capability of man to protect himself against sickness is denied, and therefore these theories, considered in a philosophical point of view, are necessarily untruths. According to these theories the germs and processes of disease find their way into the body in a manner not perceptible to the senses, or develope themselves therein in a manner that man has in none of his capabilities a warner or means of defence against them.

Moreover, these, as all dynamic theories, have the misfortune to be more or less phantasms of which one can get no clear idea, and which are set forth in learned words, since the theorists can neither give an intelligent account of the matter to themselves nor to others. Dynamis signifies strength, and we understand by "dynamic" something relating to the *higher powers*, and, very particularly, to the mainspring of all powers, *the principle of life*, of which nothing is understood. Hence it has come to pass that the word dynamic is very frequently synonymous with the idea of want of knowledge in man. More honest is it, without doubt, to confess there is a gap in science; however, it sounds more learned, and imposes on the stupid, when the space is eked out with dynamic flourishes, yet this itself shows like stupidity to those of higher intelligence. If we connect with the word dynamic the idea of that which regards the first spring of life, and the inner nature of our power, then for us human beings this is synonymous with the unexplored and unknown: in mathematics alone the word dynamic has a clear and determinate sense, when used to mark the fully investigated powers and motions of the heavenly bodies.

The physiology of man in all that relates to the inner nature, to the origin and highest energies of vitality, presents only an empty page; also on the relation of the nerves to the vital energy, and on the nature and state of the nerves, an empty page only is to be found. The physiology of man has penetrated most deeply into the laws of assimilation and secretion, and has in this province brought to light not only demonstrable principles, but has also effected a consolidation of the principles into an organic combination, into a system.

The pathology of the mediciners is founded upon the empty page of physiology, and wavers, without foundation, in the air. To it belongs as little as does to the medical therapy the claim to the name of science, and therefore the term of rationality in behalf of the medical science can only be vindicated by such physicians as have no idea of the nature of a true science.

My doctrine of disease is founded upon demonstrated and undoubted laws of physiology, and rests therefore on a solid foundation.

B.

PRACTICAL PROOF.

A PRACTICAL proof of the presence of morbific *matters* of disease has been afforded many thousand times in the results of the water-cure, inasmuch as, through the various kinds of crises in this cure, morbific matters are secreted in such a manner as to be plainly perceptible as such by the several senses. In by far the most cases, where the water cure is rightly managed and successfully employed, there arise critical eruptions and boils. That these exanthems discharge morbific matters which cause the disease, and that they consequently (with the help of water) show themselves in those persons only who have acrid and foreign matter in their bodies, is not necessary first to prove to any unprejudiced man; and no physician even has called this in question—until the discovery of the water-cure by Priessnitz. I am fully convinced that even at this day this is not really doubted by a single physician, but very many seek to persuade the public to this doubt, since the water-cure has begun to threaten the existence of the physicians. I remember very well, that seven or eight years ago many physicians contended, that if boils and eruptions appeared in a water-treatment, it were a purely accidental coincidence with the water-cure; this treatment could not be the cause of such appearances. As hydropathy afterwards became more widely extended, and as thousands of facts proved, that the application of water after the method of Vincent Priessnitz brought out boils and eruptions in the majority of secondary diseases, and also in many primary cases of disease, then indeed such a denial was no longer possible; and since then the great body of physicians have contrived another cunning in order to dispute with success the truth of the water-cure system; now they assert, it is a necessary effect of water upon the human skin, that when abundantly used, it always produces boils, even with any one perfectly healthy. I doubt indeed that any physician in the world can be so simple as really to believe this—such a belief in a disciple of the natural sciences would at least allow the presumption of a moderate degree of stupidity; but several of these gentlemen have the effrontery to endeavor to teach such like doctrines to the public, in order to keep them far as possible from the water-cure. I am almost in doubt whether to honor such an assertion with a refutation—however, for the sake of the weak it may be necessary. I refer then, to the experience of thousand fold cases, that in almost every individual case the water-cure brought out boils and eruptions,—a notorious fact, which of itself alone gives the lie to that assertion. With persons in the water-cure, that are too weak to produce a crisis and are therefore incurable, no boils or eruptions make their appearance; thousands have learned this to their deep distress. Also with persons having very weak or shattered nerves, no crises appear, when from the ignorance of their water physicians they are treated with too cold water (alas this occurs too often enough! I could mention the names of several water practitioners), and they accordingly are not cured but often injured. In the third place, no boils make their appearance in the water-cure with such persons as have no morbific matters in themselves. This is indeed a very rare occurrence, but has, however, in individual cases been amply proved. I mention among others the Norwegian, Captain Ramm, who, a Hercules in strength and health, came to Graefenberg to be cured of incipient blindness, which arose solely from over-exertion of the eyes, and not from medicinal poisoning. (Mr. Ramm was an engineer captain, had for many years been engaged in making the most delicate delineations through strongly magnifying lenses.) During a six months' cure, with the strongest application of water in douches, &c., this Hercules had not a mark of eruption or boil—indeed he was not yet cured, as in all probability he would never be perfectly. Hundreds of the Graefenberg cure-guests have also witnessed this same. A fourth class of patients in the water-cure get no boils or eruptions for this reason, because they are cured by means of strong offensively-smelling transudations; these cases are by no means seldom, and have often occurred in my practice.

The physicians, who are guilty of the above mentioned assertion, are accustomed to cite the case of washerwomen, since they get cracked hands in washing. To this we answer, that in the first place the washerwomen in winter have their hands alternately in hot and ice-cold water, which, by the long duration of the washing, is at least a mistreatment of the skin; that in the second place, corrosive stuffs such as soap and ley are here co-operating to the same end; and that in the third place, the washerwomen do not get boils nor eruptions from such injurious use of water, but cracked hands, the highest degree of brittleness and weakness even to bleeding, and the origination of holes in the flesh. This cited instance of the washerwoman, therefore, is as silly as untrue, and can at the farthest be excused only in a washerwoman.

Considered, moreover, abstractly from all experience and knowledge on the subject, it is sufficiently evident from the physiology of man, that boils and eruptions cannot be produced in perfectly healthy persons through the action of water, since water is a matter the most conceivably mild, and since boils produce a feeling always painful, and more or less acrimonious and corrosive, which can only be caused by acrid corrosive matters, or by biting animalculae which form the boil. We will comprise these boils and eruptions under the name of *Exanthems*, and then say that acrid and poisonous substances are the causes of all exanthems that are not contagious; on the other hand that living, but to the naked eye invisible, animalculae are the causes of contagious exanthems—concerning which we will treat in detail farther on.

The exanthems brought out by the water-cure vary according to the acridness of their secretions; ofttimes they are so acrid, as to eat through the linen bandages in a few weeks; always so acrid, that they cause itching, burning, and pricking. The substance of the human body may in some diseases become putrid, but never can it exert a corroding power upon the same organism from which it springs.

The causes of the not-contagious critical exanthems must therefore be foreign corroding substances, which already previous to the water-cure have lain in the diseased body, and which, through the solvent, especially the mucus dissolving power of water, are brought from the interior parts to the skin and excreted by the same. Concerning those, to the first glance apparently inexplicable, processes, by which foreign and poisonous matters can lie for years in the body without destroying it, we will in the course of this work give the detailed physiological proofs.

So much concerning the critical exanthems as instances of the materiality of the causes of disease. These exanthems, as above said, do not make their appearance with every patient in the water-cure, not even with every one that is radically cured by it, but this cure is often effected by other critical evacuations, in all of which, however, the existence of the materiality of the causes of disease comes to the plain perception of the senses. Those other critical evacuations consist in offensive smelling and viscous perspirations, in discharges of urine with unnatural smell and strong sediment, in diarrhœas, which cause a sensation of burning in the rectum, in vomiting up of matters which have a sharp medicinal poisonous taste, in acrid flow of saliva, &c.

All these crises are proofs of the existence of matters in the body, which are causing the disease.

Here the proof in relation to the offensive smelling perspirations. Firstly, there are but two substances in all nature which cause an offensive odor, namely: poisons, and everything putrifying. Secondly, the evaporations and perspirations from the skin of healthy and cleanly persons are free from smell, at least by no means bad smelling, because a healthy person exudes no poison, and because the refuse matter will be discharged from the skin of a healthy person before it has passed into putridity. Thirdly, it follows, that when the perspirations and transpirations are offensive, they are abnormal, and contain either poisonous or putrifying substance, and consequently carry matter of disease out of the body, that is, substance which was foreign to the organism.

Some readers perhaps make exception to the second position, that all perspiration even with a healthy person is offensive smelling. That, however, is not the case until it is allowed to dry up and putrify, instead of being washed off in bathing; in other words: it does not have an offensive odor in the exudation, but it gets it afterwards by its change to putridity. It is to be remembered, moreover, that I speak only of healthy and cleanly persons, and that no one can be called cleanly who does not daily wash his whole body, and that healthy persons are not to be found in the old régime or mode of living and eating. Whoever at a reasonable age has taken the water-cure until entirely cured, and afterwards adheres to the water diet, his perspiration has no trace of a disagreeable odor.

Also the viscidity of the perspiration is a proof of its containing morbid matter. This is caused by the mucous secretion, so that by this help the morbific matters may be enveloped and transported.

An argument similar to that given concerning the offensive perspirations may also be applied in respect to the flow of offensive-smelling and corrosive saliva, as also in respect to urine containing an abnormal and large sediment.

Every one acquainted with the water-cure knows that there is not a solitary instance of the cure of any chronic or acute disease without one or more of those critical evacuations mentioned in this book, and consequently not without a proof, perceptible to the senses, of the existence of material morbific matters, which cause diseases. Generally, however, there are several critical phenomena, and very often with chronic patients, they all, without exception, appear in the course of the cure one after the other.

Very often the various evacuations in the water-cure have decidedly the taste and smell of medicaments, which the patients have long since taken more than ten or twenty years ago. In vomiting crises this has often occurred in regard to the taste; in regard to the smell, these facts are realized most frequently during the critical perspirations, sometimes also from exanthems, from critical flows of urine, saliva, and alvine evacuations. It is here to be observed, that when the patients have noticed these odors arising from themselves, they have also been noticed by all others about them, so that there can be no matter of imagination in the question. Particularly the servants and attendants in water-cure establishments perceive this through their own observation, and make mention of it with astonishment.

This has occurred very frequently in my establishment, and in general, these observations have so often been made, that every one can convince himself of the truth of the same, if he questions concerning them of persons who have taken the water-cure under the care and direction of a competent water-doctor. (Under incompetent, this can not, or at most but seldom, be the case, because no crisis appears where the water-treatment is badly managed.) If desired I can point out a great number of such persons, and moreover, persons of the most unquestionable credibility.

Very often persons who have gone through a mercurial treatment years before, have again, in the water-cure, been salivated anew, which saliva tasted and smelled so decidedly of mercury, that not only the patients themselves have distinctly observed it, but also others coming in contact with them, have noticed distinctly the most marked mercurial smell. This fact proves to an infallibility, that the mercury had lain for long years as foreign matter in the body, and that it was finally in the water-cure driven out through salivation, i. e. partly through perspirations and exanthems, partly through the flow of saliva, for it is well known that we are made sensible of every scent by the olfactory nerves coming in contact with the minute but material particles of the substance smelled.

It has farthermore occurred, that by evaporating the discharges from critical boils in the water-cure, mercury and other metallic poisons have been in their chemical nature brought to light and made visible. In the various hydriatic writings are found recorded numbers of such like facts.

Thus much then for the proof philosophic and substantiated by experience of the existence of material disease-causing matters within the body. In the course of this work I will show from a number of physiological grounds, that these morbific matters not only *can* exist, but also *must* originate and exist under the false diet and false mode of cure of the old régime.

If it be conceded that morbific matters exist, and that the water-cure, by means of various kinds of crises removes them from the body, then the truth of the water-cure system and the falsity of the medical method of cure is thereby made manifest and proved. Accordingly, the mediciners dispute those facts with determination, and most commonly with all kinds of ridicule and irony. To this I here reply, from the position of the physicians themselves, firstly, that before Haller the medical theories rested upon the basis of morbific disease-causing matters, and that the most celebrated professors of medicine of that time taught this doctrine; and secondly, that for a long time after Haller, and even in the most recent times, they have admitted not only the so-called mercurial and other medicinal diseases, but also that medicinal substances remain in the body of the patient. I refer you, among others, to Dr. Kohn and Dr. Kranichstaedten, in their writings on hydropathy, and to Dr. Herr, Professor in the University at Freiburg. The latter says in his "Theory of the Operations and Effects of Medicine," page 8:—"Certain medicines, after having been in any manner applied, are found deposited in the solid parts of the body. Thus in such persons as have taken mercurial preparations, we find mercury in the brain, muscles, bones, &c. Lead is found in the liver, in the muscles, and spinal marrow. Copper deposits itself likewise in the liver. The incorporation of madder into osseous substance, is well known, and likewise that the nitrate of silver discolors the skin, and that various bitter remedies communicate their taste to the flesh." (Page 39 instances of these positions are given.) "It needs surely no farther demonstration, that, if medicines deposit themselves in the solid parts, they can only attain to it through the agency of the circulation of the blood."

Sufficiently well-known and established facts in vast number could here be cited as proofs of the deposition of medicaments and poisons in the body; among others, that workers in mercury are so interspersed with this poison, that a gold piece laid upon their tongue becomes white; that in the skeletons of old syphilitic corpses after putrefaction mercury has been found, &c. The *physicians* have treasured up all these facts for us in their writings. Accordingly, it appears certain that those physicians, who in their conversations with the lay of the profession, deny the deposition of medicaments and poisons in the solid parts of the body, in order to dispute the critical evacuations of such stuffs in the water-cure, make themselves not so much guilty of the sin of *ignorance*, as much rather of the sin of *falsehood*.

Since, now, we have proved the existence of foreign matters in the diseased body, it is still necessary to observe, that in the course of this work it will be shown, that the foreign matters in the body are not the effects, but the causes, of diseases.

I.

PROOFS FOR THE TRUTH OF

CLASSIFYING DISEASES INTO

HEALING AND DESTROYING DISEASES.

THE existence of destroying diseases (chronic diseases) needs not to be proved. Accordingly in this section we have only to do with the healing diseases (primary-acute diseases).

In the first place we borrow again a proof for the curative character of the primary diseases from the principle of optimism in philosophy.

We have above shown, that the causes of diseases already for this reason must be material, because that man with the help of his instinct can avoid material causes of disease, dynamic causes, however, not at all. When, however, despite the warnings of instinct, man takes into his body, through perverted diet and method of cure, matters of disease, then the human organism shows itself more perfect in its construction, if it at least has the relative capability of making the attempt to remove such like matters through abnormal energy and activity (through normal only it is not possible, of that see farther on), since without this endeavor and without this capability it would be immediately destroyed by such like matters, either speedily by the poisonings of the villain, or slowly by medicinal. Consequently, the existence of healing diseases may be denominated a postulate of reason, *since they do not contradict the laws of physiology, but agree with them* (particularly with the function of secretion). Still I lay no great stress upon this proof, for this reason, that the construction of man in regard to diseases has already the impress of a perfectly healthy one, since the Creator planted in him an instinct against such things as would cause disease, and for such as cure and radically heal.

If the medical method of cure were the true method, then we have implanted in man by the Creator an aversion to that which is necessary to his cure, namely, to medicine; then the creation of man is a creation entirely contrary to sense, and I, for my part, should suppose, that not the omnipotent God, but some very learned medicinal professor, or at least a Dr. Med., promotus, had prepared the human race.

In the second place we will notice several facts as proofs of the existence of healing diseases, i. e. of the healing character of the primary or acute diseases.

The most proper form of a healing disease is the pure, strong, decisive inflammation.

Experience teaches us, that none but robust persons get the real and severe inflammatory diseases, and that persons of very weak and shattered constitutions, particularly those with weak nerves, get no inflammatory diseases: also drunkards, when their health has become ruined and their nerves shattered, get no inflammatory diseases; pregnant females are less subject to those diseases than those not pregnant, having otherwise like constitutions. Well observe I speak here of acute inflammation, i. e. inflammation coming on with violent symptoms, promptly determining itself.

These statements are by no means disputed, and are well known to all physicians as well as to every observer of diseases.

From these facts alone it follows with great probability, that the inflammatory diseases are healing diseases. But still more decisive proofs of the healing character of these diseases have been afforded us by the results of the water-cure.

(1) In the water-cure treatment the inflammatory diseases are of all others the most promptly and surely cured, and in the shortest time give immense critical evacuations of morbific matters.

(2) The secondary (chronic) diseases in the water-cure pass through the following stadia:

(*a*) When a patient, with an active skin-system with strong nerves and digestive organs, consequently with strong constitution, enters upon the water-cure, having a short time previously (he can then still be strong) taken inwardly much disease-producing matter, viz. medicinal poisons: such a patient gets very soon some form of inflammatory disease, and by means thereof he drives out these morbific matters in exanthems, sweats, and other evacuations, plainly perceptible to the senses.

(*b*) When a patient, having already a very weakened and shattered constitution, pale, emaciated, or diseasedly bloated, enters upon the water-cure, he requires first a long time for the strengthening of the whole organism, for the growth of firm flesh and healthy complexion, before inflammatory symptoms appear, which thus take the same course as capitulated under *a*; and end in the elimination of perceptible morbific matters.

In a word, it is a truth established by many thousand cases, that chronic diseases are very seldom cured otherwise than by their conversion into acute, which then, with the help of the water, are followed by perceptible evacuations of the morbific matters in boils, eruptions, perspirations, diarrhœas, &c. (In water-cure establishments we generally call not only the act of elimination a crisis, but also denote thereby at the same time the abnormal excitation of the body, which precedes the discharge itself, and which almost always is attended with fever, usually with pains and inflammatory symptoms.)

From the facts presented the conclusion is satisfactory, that the primary or acute diseases are radical curative endeavors of the organism, and accordingly from their inmost nature deserve the name of healing diseases.

K.

WHAT IS POISON?

WHAT IS MEDICINE?

Observations.—1. When in this work absolute poison is mentioned, such substance is thereby intended, as, introduced into the stomach (not in the veins) in certain quantity, is fatal to life.

2. When medicine is mentioned in this work without farther epithet, then allopathic medicine is always intended.

THE SUBJECT.

The word poison may be used in a broad or limited sense; in the first it means things in general, that are deleterious to man's health; in the second, those things only which speedily produce death. The word poison may be employed in the figurative or in the strict literal sense; in the first it signifies the pernicious and fatal influences of the external world upon man, whatever may be their manner of operation, whether the chemical, the physical, the mechanical, or the moral. We take in our treatise the word poison always in the strict literal sense, which regards purely the chemical operation of a substance on the human body. When we understand mechanical or dynamic poisons, we will always attach the corresponding epithet to the word.

Poison, in the strict sense of the word, or strong poison, is a substance, which, taken in the human stomach in a suitable quantity, is fatal to the life of every person without distinction, if this substance be not again ejected by vomiting immediately. We must set some limit to the term "suitable quantity," which may be variously selected. The most natural measure for "suitable quantity" appears at first sight to be such a quantity as is equal to an ordinary meal. However, with all stronger poisons it is an absolute impossibility to take such a quantity into the stomach, and consequently we will take the second natural measure, namely, the quantity of one ordinary mouthful, and say, poison in the strict sense of the word is a substance, which taken into the stomach, to the quantity of an ordinary mouthful, causes death to every person without distinction, if it is not removed again by vomiting. It is evident, that for the attainment of a more determinate boundary between poison in the stricter and broader sense, a fixed weight should be substituted for mouthful, which we here omit, because here the *result* of the demarcation is by no means of importance, but simply the *demonstration* of the demarcation.

Poison, in the broader sense of the word, or the class of milder poisons, is a substance, which, by its chemical effect on any person, even the healthiest, produces decided marks of disease, if the substance be taken in the quantity of an ordinary meal.

The above given explanations relate to the absolute

poisons, and in this work we understand by poison, without farther epithet, always that which is for man absolutely poisonous.

What is called relative poison, i. e. substances which are wholesome to the healthy, but partly through chemical effect, partly from the quantity thereof, or quantitative effect, are deleterious to sick and weak persons, and even fatal, that belongs not in the least here, and must be entirely excluded from the elucidation of absolute poison.

That, which to man is absolutely poisonous, is again relatively poisonous to other classes of organisms.

In regard to the entire creation there is no absolute poison, but in regard to every individual species, and e. g. in regard to the human race, there is a mass of absolute poisons, and we treat here of men only.

Whoever, in the definition of poisons, in the broader sense of the word, or the milder class of poisons, given by me, will accuse it of vacancy and falsity of illustration, because there is no marked boundary given between poison and non-poison, to him I reply two-fold, viz. in the first place, I repeat, that a determined absolute measure or weight could be easily substituted for the relative measure of an ordinary meal, that then the demarcation would be stricter, that here we are not in the least concerned with the results of the demarcation, but only with the demonstration of it. In the second place, I reply to such an one that important and undisputed word often spoken by me, that nowhere in nature and in objective truth are to be found marked limits between different species and different classes, and consequently in the reality, there are no species and classes in the strict sense of these words.

It is not possible between poison and non-poison to draw a sharp and ever determinate boundary taken from nature, but only a conventional boundary. It is just as little possible to draw anywhere else in nature a sharp and true line of demarcation, e. g. between trees and shrubbery. If, therefore, any one says there is no poison, because there is no sharp boundary line between poison and non-poison, he must necessarily also say, there are no trees, because there is no fixed boundary between a tree and sapling; he must also say, there is no black and no white race of men, because there is no sharply marked boundary between both races; he must even say there is nothing, because nowhere in nature are there sharply marked limitations.

As between all species there are unobservable transitions and connecting links, so also between poison and non-poison there must be a copula, a point of indifference, and this intermediate substance must under certain circumstances, be pernicious, under others, uninjurious and even wholesome. In regard to man, table salt and spices constitute these transition substances; namely, unmixed with other things these spices are injurious, mixed with certain articles of food, they are at least not so in all countries.

The mixture of salt and of spices with articles of food leads us to the chapter upon the mixture of relative poisons with other articles, and to the question of their injuriousness in the mixture. The answer to this can be easily and definitely given, viz. that substance, which taken unmixed and pure, produces symptoms of disease, is then uninjurious in its mixture with other articles of food, if its taste in the mixture is plainly perceptible, and still to a healthy man agreeable. (By healthy men, I understand only such, from whose diet all artificial, all poisonous, and all imported stimulants from foreign zones, are excluded.) If we add this elucidation to the above-given definition of poisons, we have found in it a demarcation, which also allots to the transition substances, salt and spices, their appointed place.

The next question in the determination of the term "poison" is, whether those substances, which in a specified quantity produce partly speedy death, partly speedily ensuing symptoms of disease, also still absolutely produce pernicious effects, and consequently still then remain absolute poison, when they are taken in smaller quantity. Logic, as well as physiology, reply in the affirmative. But before we proceed, we must observe that this question has led us imperceptibly into the territory of medicine, and that before replying to the same with logical and physiological reasons, we must give the definition of the term "medicine."

What is medicine? The word medicine, or medicament, signifies, in its literal translation, a means of cure for diseases. In this broad and original sense we do not accept the word here, as also in general it is no more used in such a sense: e. g. no one calls the sympathetic method of treatment a medical method, and one calls the sympathist a mediciner. The word has only retained this broad signification in figurative language, which, however, is excluded from our treatise.

The words "medicine" and "medicament," in the limited and modern sense, are those articles, the trade in, and preparation of, which, are the peculiar privilege of the apothecaries, comprising all the various kind of poisons, or by far the greater part. There is not a solitary poison but what is administered by physicians as a means of cure for disease, and that with the permission of government. Thus I am legally in my good right when I call medicine poison, and I will now show that in this expression I am also in physiological right.

Since I, in my hydriatic writings, have with determination upbraided the physicians with the use of poison and of poisoning their patients (I mean of course, a poisoning through error not from intention), they seek, through all kinds of excuses and justifications, to convince the people of the untruth of the accusation; are, however, very unfortunate in their logic, and take good care not to come out publicly in print with such pretended rectifications of my writings and views, to which I have invited the gentlemen as urgently as courteously.

The first excuse of the mediciners consists in the assertion that there is nowhere poison; anything might become poisonous under certain circumstances, to individual persons. This latter is perfectly true with the relative poisons in regard to the human race; but it is perfectly false with the absolute poisons, of which I have just shown that the definition and determination thereof may be settled in like manner as with all other terms. In this proof I have limited myself to the introduction solely of poisons into the stomach; it needs scarcely be said, that we could just as well and in like manner, with the introduction of various stuffs through the skin, or a wound into the circulation, set a determined measure or weight, which is sufficient to destroy any human being, as a definitive mark for the term poison. Thus, therefore, is the excuse of the physicians foiled, viz. that there is no decided poison, and that every article may become a poison to the health of individual persons, thus making the absolute poisons relative, and the relative poisons absolute at their pleasure.

The second article of justification of the physicians consists in the assertion that the quantity only of any substance makes it a poison, and that the same substance is poison when used in great quantity, but by no means poison, but a means of health, i. e. a means of cure, when taken in smaller quantities.

First, a word against the logical falsity and impossibility of this assertion. If a substance, which in a certain quantity produces death, be given in a smaller quantity, then every à priori conclusion, according to the laws of logic, must come to this determination, that this substance in a less quantity exerts a less powerful effect, accordingly, causes slow death. All analogies from the sciences of chemistry and physiology speak in the most decided terms for this, my conclusion, and against that of the mediciners. In the kingdoms of chemistry and physiology the law obtains that by reduction of the quantity of the matter, first, the disposition thereof remains the same, and second, the chemical effect is, in like ratio, diminished; but this chemical effect always continues to be a corresponding and never a contrary-disposed effect. We may, therefore, with a full right pronounce the assertion that the chemical effect of smaller doses of poison is a contrary one to the chemical effect of larger doses of the same, a physiological and chemical untruth, because this assertion contradicts all known laws of physiology and chemistry. This assertion lacks every foundation, even the shadow of a foundation, and is purely extracted from air.

Directly below we will take up and disprove this assertion from specially physiological grounds, and first make the observation that, premising the truth of this false principle, it ought necessarily to be verified by the instinct of man and beast; but experience teaches the contrary, namely, that the instinct of man as well as of beast exhibits the most utter abhorrence to these small doses of poison, which do not cause instantaneous death, and which are administered by the physicians as intended means of cure, which abhorrence deters them from taking such remedies. (Hereafter I will show that the admonitions of instinct of a pure man of nature, not only are unerring, but are absolutely necessary to the continuation and propagation of our race upon the earth.)

We arrive at a physiological disproval of the above-mentioned assertion of the physicians, when we show the physiological laws and processes through which poisons exert their destroying power on the animal, and particularly on the human, organism.

The human body is indeed no chemically simple body, but it is, when in a state of health, a physiologically simple body, i. e. there should be, when it is healthy, no matter in it, which offers resistance to its power of appropriation, and thence becomes foreign matter, and throws hindrances in the way of the exercise of the physiological functions of the organism. Everything, which in proper fineness and respective fluidity is introduced into the stomach, or for a length of time kept in contact with the skin, or a wounded part, is incorporated either partially or wholly into part and parcel of the body, and is carried, through the circulation of the blood, into all, even the deepest and remotest, parts of the human body.

There is no substance which, introduced into the body through an incision in a large or small vein, can be assimilated by the organic power of that body. Every substance, therefore, which in such manner gets into the body is foreign to the same. The veins have no organs of assimilation.

With the human skin it is otherwise ; that organ is capable of digesting two substances, viz. air and water,—but all else that gets in the body through absorption of the skin, cannot be assimilated by the skin, and is consequently foreign and deleterious to the constitution.

The strongest and most comprehensive digestive and assimilating power resides in the stomach and intestines, and for this reason these organs have been called exclusively the digestive organs.

From the specified construction of the veins, it follows that all whatsoever is directly introduced into them through an opening in them, is poison to the human body, at least in the broader sense of the word.

From the constitution of the human skin it follows that with the exception of air and water, all fluid or half fluid substances, kept for a length of time in contact with it, are poison to the human body, either in the broader or stricter sense of the word. I mention this particularly, for this reason, to prevent the objection urged by the doctors against my exposition, inasmuch as they might say that water also could become a poison, if it were introduced into a vein. In the elucidation of absolute poison, the argument can only concern those substances which introduced into the stomach have a fatal and sickening effect. Hence, the objection taken from those substances, which introduced immediately into the veins are absolutely pernicious, is one that of itself falls to pieces and originates in a men.al confusion.

What substances can the healthy stomach digest?

The only infallible and all-comprising answer that can here be given, is taken from the intimations of instinct, and purports thus: all those things for which the healthy unpoisoned palate has appetite. This answer is absolutely infallible, and proves the injuriousness of all medicaments.

Do we inquire as to the chemical nature of those substances, which agree with or cause disgust to the human palate, we can give no other answer so unerring and exclusive.

However, there are three conditions, that determine the digestibility of substances as far as the animal man is concerned.

First, These substances must not be spoiled, i. e. have become putrid. When they are so, and are still eaten, they pass as putrid juices into the body, and are consequently foreign and injurious matter.

Second, These substances must be of such a nature that they can be readily dissolved into infinitely minute particles by the gastric juice diluted with water. Consequently, all substances that resist this dissolution, as for instance stones, earths, and metals, are indigestible.

Third, The digestible substances must be less acid and weaker than the gastric juice of the consumer, because in entire nature the law prevails that the stronger vitality overpowers and appropriates the weaker. This law is of exceeding great importance, and in consequence of this law the digestive juice of man must possess a very high degree of sharpness, if he is to have the capability of digesting a vast number of various substances. This sharpness of the digestive juice is produced partly by the secretions of the glands of the stomach itself, still more, however, by the bile discharged into the duodenum. Man should, therefore, eat nothing that is sharper than the digestive juice, and instinct directs man in this respect with perfect safety, since all uncorrupted nerves of taste experience from such sharper substances a very disagreeable burning and stinging sensations.

The first class of indigestible substances forms the intermediate link between poison and non-poison, and consists consequently of relative poisons.

The second class consists of absolute poisons, and comprises partly those poisons which toxicology denominates astringent poisons, partly somewhat of those that are called mechanical poisons, and operate mostly through constipation of the small vessels.

The third, by far the most important and dangerous class of poisons, consists of those by the toxicology classed under the head of "corrosive" and "narcotic" poisons, and they operate fatally through their corrosive and narcotic power, against which the organism reacts with mucous secretions, and accumulations of blood (inflammation).

The most deadly poisons of the corrosive and narcotic class are administered by the physicians as remedies for all violent symptoms of disease, which for the most part are of primary, sometimes also of secondary nature, as for instance, violent cramps belong to the severe secondary symptoms of diseases. The corrosive poisons are not administered by physicians in cases of lingering atonic disease, but only narcotic poisons in dilutions and weak preparations, in opposition to which the narcotic poisons, when administered for violent symptoms, are given in an undiluted, mostly concentrated and sublimated form.

The corrosive and narcotic poisons form the drastic medicaments; all these poisons, when not in a manner diluted, as indeed the homœopaths prepare them, but the allopaths never, have a much sharper substance than the gastric juice; consequently, their digestion, even in the smallest allopathic doses, is an impossibility; consequently, absolute poison never ceases, through smallness of the dose, to be poison, can never be a means of cure, because it can never be digested.

Absolute poison loses, through smallness of the allopathic doses, none of its disgusting and horrible taste to the palate, it is thus marked as poison by the instinct as much as by the laws of physiology, and by experimental chemistry.

The physicians, who, for the vindication of their profession and to parry my attacks, would much too willingly declare the poisons administered by themselves for non-poisons, and maintain that a substance is poison only according to its quantity, allege the inverted argument, that wholesome substances taken to excess, may also become poison. To this I reply: first, The unconditional inversion of a position is well known to be logically unallowable, and is therefore a logic blunder, which bears on its face the stamp of falseness.

Second, Substances in themselves wholesome, exert, through their excess, an injurious effect upon *healthy* persons not *chemically* but *mechanically*, through too violent distension, and consequently succeeding relaxation of the over-burdened organs. Therefore, these substances, taken to excess, belong not to the chemical but to the mechanical poisons, and thus this whole pretence of the physicians rests upon a change of the signature of classification, and arises from a mental confusion, and is entirely false.

Third, Substances of themselves wholesome and difficult of digestion, may become injurious through their chemical effect upon diseased digestive organs, because the organs are not possessed of normal strength; therefore, these substances may be to them *relative* poisons: in this chapter, however, we are not speaking of *relative* poisons, as oft observed, but of absolute poisons; thus this objection rests also upon a confusion of ideas. Granted, however, that this is not the case, then this objection still neither says nor proves anything in favor of the false position, namely, that poisonous substances, from minuteness of the dose, lose their poisonous qualities, and assume a contrary quality, and become curative remedies for mankind. It is very clearly evident, that substances difficult of digestion, for which the whole strength of a healthy stomach is requisite, cannot be digested by a weak and diseased stomach, and, therefore, may be relative poison to the possessor of the diseased stomach. But the inversion of this argument, namely, that substances or poisons, which the healthy person cannot digest, the sick person shall be able to digest, and that such substances may become true remedies, is a logical and physiological untruth.

From the foregoing results of this treatise on poison the correctness of the definition given by me proves itself; every substance that passes from the stomach and bowels into the human body without being digested, is at least relative poison; every substance, however, that is by man absolutely indigestible, is absolute poison.

In this definition we have the rationale of the manner in which poisons exert their evil effect upon the organism, viz. in this wise, that they remain as foreign matter in the organism.

Since that, in the foregoing, I have proved the existence of absolute poisons, and that substances do not lose their poisonous effects through diminution of the dose, I must say a few words upon the mixture and the combination of poisons.

(1) *Mixture of poisons.*—In this question, whether, in the strong mixture of poisonous substances with wholesome, the poisonous lose their deleterious effect, and, consequently are divested of their poison, Homœopathy only can come under consideration, since Allopathy never admixes its poisons to such a degree, that they lose their poisonous effect, which can be proved by chemical tests, as well as by the taste which they bear; also, it is by no means the purpose of allopathy to reduce their medicinal poisons so considerably by dilution, as to cause them to lose their natural and chemical effect; it aims rather to *increase* these effects by sublimation and concentration.

Homœopathy, on the contrary, dilutes its medicines to such a degree, that neither the art of chemistry, nor the nerves of taste, can discover any of the original poisonous effects of the administered medicaments. For this purpose it makes use of water, and that is the only substance which, by its very copious admixture, can perhaps deprive poison of all its pernicious influences, and certainly removes these effects, in so far that they are no more perceptible, either to the senses or the chemical art

For my part, I do not venture to decide upon it, whether the absolute abstraction of the strength of the poisons is effected by such dilution ; if such a possibility exist, it is thus rendered possible only by admixture with water, and the least so, by admixture with solid substances. One thing, however, is certain, viz. that such an abstraction of the poison, through the agency of water, is possible only when the uncorrupted palate can no more perceive the most remote taste of the poison in the commixture. In the homœopathic doses after the decillionth dilution, the slightest taste of the poison is no more perceptible, and consequently, I believe that such doses are absolutely divested of their poisonous influences on the human body, and for this reason have always had the most profound respect for this method of cure, in comparison with the allopathic, and looked upon it as a blessing to the human race.

After having refuted all the arguments that have as yet come to my hearing, adduced by physicians, against my complaint, that they treat with poison and poison their patients, I must, in conclusion, say a word

(2) *Concerning the combination of poisons,* because from that source also, the physicians have endeavored a vindication of cure with poisons.

A poison, combined with a non-poisonous body or substance, is such an one as can be obtained or freed from the combination only by a chemical transformation of the substance with which it is combined. *The combined poisons are free from all effective poisonous power or influence, and hence receive their name, because their powers are bound up.* Accordingly, poison combined or bound up, is to the human organism decidedly a non-poison, since neither the nerves of taste are capable of detecting it, nor the other organs experience any evil effect therefrom. In my opinion, the expression "combined poison" is one very unhappily selected, and originated in chemical error. Combined poison is not at all present as poison in the combination, *but in the combination substances are present, which, by means of chemical processes, can be converted into poisons.* Thus, for instance, Prussian blue can be unbound or fabricated from the human blood through chemical processes (however, in exceedingly small quantity), from most fruits by fermentation and distillation, alcohol, from the basis of water and air (viz. from hydrogen, nitrogen, and oxygen), several powerful poisons. In these substances themselves there is not the least poison present, but only constituents that can be converted into poison.

When, therefore, physicians adduce arguments in behalf of their method of cure with *free* poisons from this subject of *combined* poisons, there lies, also, again at the bottom of it, a perversion of terms, which no one should make himself guilty of, who has studied chemistry.

From the presence of combined poison in the blood, in elements, &c., the physicians could only justify a treatment with combined poisons, i. e. with substances without any effect. But it is notorious that the physicians administer their poisons in a free uncombined state only.

As the mechanical poisons, to which belong pieces of glass, points of needles, and the like, are excluded from this chapter on chemical poisons, I was obliged, in accordance with my pathology, to exclude the contagious poisons also, because they, as will be shown hereafter, belong, likewise, to the class of mechanical poisons. These contagious poisons consist, as I shall show in the proper place, of small invisible animalculæ, mostly mites (as in the itch), which increase by propagation and engender the symptoms of disease, the contagious boils and eruptions by their eating and gnawing.

Now, I think all false arguments, by which physicians endeavor to deny their use of poison, have been refuted and exhibited in their entire falsity. Should such arguments of more recent invention come to my knowledge, I will not fail to subject them to criticism.

I.

OF THE EFFECTS OF COLD WATER

UPON THE HUMAN ORGANISM IN GENERAL.

PRELIMINARY REMARKS.—The word cold, as it appertains to water in its general relation to man, comprises a scale of many various degrees. It cannot be much colder than 32° Fah., because at that point it becomes ice; ascending on the scale, it must, in regard to the human body, be called cold in common parlance, so long as it does not reach the blood-warmth, i. e. 100° Fah., in contradiction to which, it becomes warm water as soon as it exceeds 100° Fah.

In the water-cure system, however, we stand in need of designations for smaller divisions of the scale. Water, warmer than 77° Fah. is never employed according to the system of Vincent Priessnitz. We will call all water under 55° Fah. cold; all water between 55° and 77° Fah. tepid, and all water above 100° warm.

SUBJECT.

In investigations upon the effects of water under 77° Fah. there come consequently into consideration, first, the degree of cold, and second, the chemical composition of the water.

(7) At a very low temperature and by long continuance it has a fatal effect upon the human organism by the merely absolute abstraction of warmth. At a more moderate temperature and in shorter duration, it effects a partial abstraction of warmth, which is again restored to a proper balance by the organism conducting blood to the refrigerated part. An abnormally strong determination of blood to this part is necessary to the restoration of this balance.

The first effect of the cold is, therefore, repulsion of the blood from the part of the body subjected thereto, the contra-operation of the organism is increase of heat in the refrigerated part; this contra-operation is often called the after-effect of the cold.

If one subjects any one part much oftener than the rest of the body to a short exposure to cold, the current of the blood must by degrees be directed to this part more especially, and become accustomed to the direction. The part or organ thus affected must be well nourished and warmed by the thus increased to and fro current of the blood. For the law holds good, that the contra-effect or reaction always far exceeds in duration the first effect of a short application of cold, and exceeds it also in energy, if the organism be vigorous. Moreover, with persons of strong nerves the reaction is so much the more energetic the greater the difference of temperature between the body and the cold, and the more sudden the transition from warm to cold.

Hence it follows, that in cold we have in our power a means to the voluntary regulation of the circulation of the blood, and that where the cold is most applied, thither also the energies of the organism, blood and heat, betake themselves the most.

But the reaction against the cold of the air is in proportion to the action thereof, much slighter than the reaction against the cold of the water, because water from its constituent parts exercises a much more decomposing action upon the skin than the air does, and hence a higher reaction, and more increased press of blood must be produced in the part cooled with water, than in the part cooled by the air.

Delicate persons, and those inclined to rheumatism, cannot for this reason be hardened by the cold of the air alone, but only in conjunction with the cold of water. Persons with shattered nerves cannot endure any considerable degree of cold, and on this account water much less cold must be used by them, than by healthy persons. Air, water, and cold, are called in the favorite words of the doctors stimulating remedies ; here these words are indeed used in a right application, but in a measure drawn from the surface, since in them the process of stimulation is not at the same time expressed ; the words : means of producing reaction would be at all events words of clearer signification. But we will here let the expression stimulating remedies remain.

If the stimulating remedies are to answer the purpose of strengthening permanently individual organs or parts of the body, they must introduce nothing into the body, that is incapable of being assimilated, and therefore always burden the organ upon which they are directed more and more, instead of relieving it, and at length ruin it completely. Daily experience proves this to satisfaction, and physiology explains the phenomenon in the clearest manner. For when the parts of the body, that are to be strengthened, are gradually burdened more and more with such substances, as they cannot convert into their own kind, and which are settled in them as foreign and forsooth as acrid and therefore inimical matters, a disturbance of the circulation of the blood, and a still greater disturbance of the secretions is thereby induced. Alcohol is one of the chief stimulants of the physicians; this acknowledged poison is absolutely indigestible, is absolutely foreign to the chemical nature of the human body, and gradually ruins the organ into which it is introduced entirely by its sharp poisonous energy. By washing weak parts of the body with spirits, by the application of French brandy, especially to the eyes, in short by the use of all remedies containing alcohol, the organs treated therewith become gradually more and more weakened.

The invigoration of the general organism is alone possible by the expulsion of morbific matter, and by wholesome nutrition.

The invigoration of an individual organ, i. e. the elevation of it above other organs, or an alteration of the proportion which the organs bear to one another, is only possible through the use of remedies which produce reaction, and since all medicinal stimulants, as above shown, event in time in the poisoning and depression of the organ stimulated by them, an alteration in the proportion of the strength of the functions and organs to one another is only possible by means of the stimulants of nature, air, water, and the more or less cold combined therewith.

(2) The *chemical constitution* of water in reference to its power of operation upon the human organism has al-

ready been considered in the sections A. and B. in their main points of interest, and consequently but few words upon the subject will be here required.

Water is the only dissolvent in nature, as many physicians, to wit, Hufeland in his Makrobiotique, have admitted. Water is, moreover, the only liquid in nature capable of flowing in drops—all such other liquids consist of water and of more or less minute solid particles. These other liquids have therefore the general dissolvent power in less degree than water, because in the first place the best part of this solvent power is already exhausted upon the solid particles therein dissolved, and because in the second place these solid particles are of themselves obstacles to the solution of other substances, and obstacles to the penetration of the fluid into the most minute spaces and interstices.

In the foregoing we have seen, that the human body unceasingly excretes the refuse matter of its own essence, and requires to be supplied with fresh substance for its support by means of assimilation. Both functions can proceed in a normal and perfect manner only by inward and outward use of water.

The nutrition of the body is aided in a double manner by water, viz. first because the chyle is promptly and perfectly dissolved into its minutest particles by the water taken into the stomach, which is necessary to its absorption in the ileum and jejunum. Second, oxygen gas, which is requisite to the formation of solid matter from the blood, the last act of nutrition, is offered to all, even the smallest and most remote parts of the body, by the water taken into the stomach, which is always absorbed by the above named intestines, and thus, before it passes off, makes its way through the veins and through the heart; oxygen gas is, indeed, taken in the blood in part through the process of respiration, but it must be also in part drawn from the water, which is drunk, as in the case of diseases, when frequently an abnormal quantity of oxygen is demanded in certain parts of the body for the purpure of cure.

(*b*) Water is also just as indispensable to the excretory functions. By virtue of its pure fluidity it penetrates the whole body, and by virtue of the hydrogen it contains, it is the means by which the organism converts solid matter into liquid, and thus makes it capable of excretion.

Therefore water, by virtue of its chemical constituent parts, affords the best means for the nutrition of the body, and for replacing waste matter, and all substance which may be wanting in its individual organs, and it affords the only medium for the removal of matters burdensome to the body, whether they be solid or fluid. When it is taken into consideration, that *cold water* is the best means for the correction of the circulation, and of the disturbed balance among the individual functions and organs,—we are compelled to draw thence the indubitable conclusion, that water is the most important and most worthy of regard of all curative means. The other means of cure are fresh air, exercise, wholesome nourishment, and healthy occupation; without being combined with these other assistant remedies, water can effect nothing; but if the organic strength of the person is insufficient, then all together are useless.

M.

THE PRIMARY OR HEALING DISEASES.

I.

THE MANNER IN WHICH PRIMARY DISEASES IN GENERAL ARISE.

THE human body exists under an unceasing labor of excretion and fresh formation of humor, flesh, and bony substance. In the course of several years the body of a healthy person is so completely renovated, that of its whole substance, even to the minutest atom, nothing of the old is any more present. Physiologists differ very widely as to the length of time required for complete renovation, variously assuming it from two to seven years.

As the body does not possess the capability of holding itself at rest in one and the same state, but is under the necessity of constant renewal and excretion of waste matter; the conditions for the appeasement of these wants must be guaranteed to it. Adequate aliment is necessary to the renovation of the body, and to the normal undisturbed healthy excretion of waste matter daily contact with air and water is indispensable, in order that these elements may exercise their dissolvent power on the skin, and absorb from the body through the pores that which must be removed from it, if it is not to become burdened with stagnant matter and thus sicken.

When the conditions of health are for a length of time vouchsafed only imperfectly and partially to the body, it loses gradually the normal energy of all its functions. If, then, while in such a state, the general tone of the system being thus depressed, an extraordinary attack from any side whatsoever be directed against the body or one of its organs, it cannot otherwise react and defend itself, than by an extraordinary abnormally heightened exertion of its powers, that is, by some *primary disease.*

There are but two kinds of diseases to which the *healthy* person in the air and water diet is still exposed; first, the epidemic diseases, and those peculiar to certain climates, produced by corruption of the atmosphere; second, contagious exanthematous diseases, small pox, &c.

All other diseases are the result of the ordinary perverted mode of diet, and false method of cure.

II.

HYDRIATIC CURE OF THE PRIMARY DISEASES.

THE abnormal morbid exertions of an organism to expel morbific matters are the signs of reaction or the symptoms of acute disease. These, the water-physician assists and promotes, and attains thereby a certain and radical cure, the object of these symptoms—through diarrhœa and vomiting in stomach and digestive complaints, and in all others through perspirations, rashes, boils, and critical urinations. Farther on, the special processes will be shown, with citation of instances.

A state of health far superior to that enjoyed before the disease is the consequence of every primary disease cured with water. General or local weakness, or otherwise after-pains of any kind, never ensue; after a few days, he that is cured with water, can undergo labors and fatigue with increased energies and enhanced vigor, far surpassing what he enjoyed before the disease.

III.

MEDICINAL CURE OF THE SAME DISEASES.

When poison is administered to a body which is making that acute struggle to cure itself, it must divert a part of its powers of reaction and turn them against this poison, in order to expel it by vomiting and evacuation, or surround it with mild mucous juices quickly formed for the occasion, that it may not corrode and injure the body. The energies and juices, which the organism calls forth in this manner to surround the medicine with mucus, must be withdrawn from the struggle which it is holding with the original enemy—viz. the disease. From this cause a moderation in the symptoms ensues, and when the poison is administered in suitable quantity, and with proper repetition, the organism must call forth all its energies to cope this dangerous enemy, desist entirely from its original curative struggle, and thus the symptoms subside. Then, according to the doctors' manner of speaking, the disease is cured. If the body thus treated afterwards endeavors anew to cure itself, and calls up these symptoms again, they consider it a relapse into the disease, and poison it anew, until either death or disappearance of the symptoms ensues.

In most primary cases the same effect may be attained by copious blood-lettings as by means of the poisons. These draughts upon the vital principle must be regulated always according to the strength of the patient, to deprive him of the strength and ability required for an acute ardent struggle, whereupon the disease is "cured."

Instinct tells every unfortunate one, who has thus been poisoned and leeched under the old system of cure, that his doctor grossly errs when he calls him "cured;" instinct says, that in his body something foreign, inimical, has taken up its quarters, and every one of these deplorable beings requires a long time for the re-collection of his scattered energies, and must pursue an anxious and painful regimen. Instead of which, every one treated from the commencement with water may, in a few days after any primary disease, undertake whatever he will, eat as much and of what he likes, go out and in both at evening and night, according to his pleasure. In the hydriatic treatment it very rarely occurs that the patient even loses his appetite for any number of days during the disease.

From the demonstrated nature of the effects of poisons it appears, that in many cases it must be matter of small moment which kind of poison is selected, that it depends much more upon the quantity of the dose, which is designed to cripple the organism to a sufficient degree, without killing it outright. Experience confirms this to a certainty. Even the apparently so peculiar effect of the so called specifics rests upon nothing else than their general poisonous effect. For instance, China cures the intermitting fever, and was for a long time supposed to be the only specific for that complaint; in later times it has been discovered that belladonna and arsenic suppress the fever much more effectually, because they are more injurious poisons. In this manner many diseases can be cured allopathically by one and the same poison.

There are, however, many exceptions at hand, viz. in all those primary diseases, which have their symptoms exclusively in one organ or system of the body, the suppression of these symptoms and of the healing-struggle must be effected most promptly, and with the proportionately smallest dose, if that poison be employed which produces with healthy persons in that same organ contrary symptoms of disease (contraria contrariis).

From these grounds it becomes evident whence it is that almost every physician has his favorite poison, with which he cures almost all complaints, the one mercury, the other opium, &c., viz. every physician, by various experiments with his favorite medicine, arrives at the result, that it in most cases accomplishes the same as that medicament prescribed by the "science" for every different case, and thus each one thinks he has found the universal medicine.

For the physician, mercury is indisputably the most advantageous poison that can be used in most diseases, for this reason, that this poison developes its injurious effects the most tardily, and consequently, in the opinion of the poisoned, releases the doctor from all blame for the complaints which afterwards appear. Thus mercury has recently become the most favorite medicine of physicians, and it may not be long ere we shall behold children born with salivation and caries of their bones! so mercurially diseased to the very root even is this European race.

When, in future, "medicine" is made mention of in this work, allopathy is always intended thereby.

IV.

THE NORMAL STOMACH.

In our stomach-poisoned European race we have scarcely a correct idea of the constitution of a stomach possessing normal strength and health.

The stomach of every man of nature possesses the following qualities: first, great power of dilation and contraction; he can fast several days without injury to his health; and vice versâ, he can take nourishment sufficient for several days at *one* meal without "indigestion."

Further, if poisons or absolutely indigestible substances find their way into his stomach, he vomits them out again with great energy and ease; if it is surfeited with food beyond its utmost power of digestion, it likewise relieves itself by vomiting. For this reason, indigestion, or even death, is quite impossible from the most beastly surfeit. In the temperate and frigid climates, the frequent use of fat is wholesome to the healthy stomach,* and necessary to the healthfulness of the general digestion. These qualities the stomach, in the water-diet, retains until death; without the daily use of water no one can retain

* The diseased and medicine-poisoned stomach must eschew fat, even in the commencement of the water-cure, until it has become much strengthened.

perfect healthfulness of stomach and vigor of body to the end of his life.

Cold water, from the reaction which it produces, gives to the stomach that permanent high degree of warmth, without which the perfect energy of this organ is impossible. The healthy stomach of the water-drinker craves frequent and copious draughts of water, to cool and refresh the elevated warmth of the stomach, and it is these coolings also, which serve to reproduce and maintain it. On the contrary, a stomach accustomed to warm and stimulating artificial drinks, craves always at certain periods this artificial warming, whereby its condition of normal warmth becomes more and more depressed. Such a stomach is faint in the morning until it gets its coffee, and thereby its "tone." To the stomach of the water-drinker the feeling of languidness is quite unknown.

Water only is capable of keeping the stomach and bowels during the whole course of life pure and free from all sliming, i. e. from becoming coated with mucus and slimy matter.

Water operates very stimulating by means of its constituent parts, oxygen gas and hydrogen gas, which gases are the true spirits of life and fire.

Water is, directly and immediately through its dissolvent power, the most effective of all promoters of digestion. Lay a piece of raw meat in wine, brandy, beer, broth, or other soup, or even in stomach bitters, and observe which best macerates it, these fluids or water. One might almost be ashamed of being compelled to speak of things with which every cook is acquainted, and from which every child's understanding can make the conclusion and application. But the stupidity of the old régime has so filled the people with prejudices, that one must prove at large the most simple truths. If all my arguments do not yet suffice you, then cast your eyes about you into the kingdom of life—have you ever heard of a wild animal afflicted with the stomach disease, unless it were a lapdog, which takes its coffee and soup at the table with its mistress? Does some one say to me, that man is not a beast? to him I reply, that as far as concerns his bodv he is as other animals.

The Graefenberg water-cure heals the most wretched stomach, and elevates it to such a degree of energy as is seldom to be found with even the persons so-called healthy of the old régime. I am acquainted with several who have, from the depths of chronic stomach disease, attained through the water-cure, such a strength of stomach that the heartiest meal never troubles them, and they observe no difference between light and heavy foods, that they can eat even fat pastry, and moreover, fat by the spoonful, without feeling the least uncomfortable sensations thereafter.

The Graefenberg diet, whereby so great results are obtained, is in its details mostly the contradiction of the old régime. Water and boiled milk the only drinks, the foods cooled or cold, excluding all artificial stimulants, everything bitter, everything from foreign zones, and most especially all medicinals. We perceive that this diet is the nearest possible approach to nature, to the diet of a man of nature.

The wholesomeness of water for the stomach has just before been shown. Here still a word upon the wholesomeness of the most possibly simple, and not piquant, not exciting foods.

The digestion, the assimilation of foreign matter into the human body, is possible only when the gastric juice possesses more sharpness and higher vital power than the chyle, that is, than the food taken into the stomach after having undergone the process of mastication. Hence, it follows that the simple aliments are easier of digestion than the sharp, spicy, or piquant. However, this simpleness must not be carried to that degree which produces in the uncorrupted instinct a feeling of unpleasant vacancy. Man undoubtedly requires more piquant aliments than most beasts; he resembles the fruit-eating beasts, and needs, therefore, especially aliments which contain much saccharine matter. Entirely foreign to the man of nature are the sharp, burning spices, the sharp bitternesses, and most of all the foreign alcoholic drinks.

The uncorrupted instinct affords a correct discrimination between the wholesomeness and unwholesomeness of foods, especially the instinct of a child which is born of healthy parents, and has never been compelled to swallow anything which is to him disagreeable or loathsome, or excites in him feelings of disgust and horror.

The apparent promotion of digestion by means of stimulants and piquant articles of food, much salt and spice, rests upon a misunderstanding easily detected. These articles excite the salivary and stomach glands to a momentary increased secretion of juices, and this abnormal reaction to carry off and overcome the stimulating remedies awakens a feeling of false hunger; but they do not strengthen, they weaken. The stimulating remedies are to the stomach precisely what the spur is to the worn-out horse. Will any one be so stupid as to believe, the spur strengthens the horse?

V.

PRIMARY STOMACH DISEASES IN GENERAL.

It is extremely seldom that we find chronic conditions of disease of a simple nature; the secondary complaints are rather a compound affection frequently of many organs, generally of several at a time.

Patients, in particular, afflicted with secondary diseases, are rarely found with healthy digestion, because the stomach and bowels are quite naturally those organs, which are the first and most affected and injured by the poisons which may be taken.

Stomach diseases are not only so numerous as physicians suppose, but still more so; for many diseases have their roots in the digestive organs, and their symptoms in other organs; consequently, the doctors exercise their art on these other functions, because they always strive to suppress the symptoms of disease.

For these reasons, that the stomach governs all other organs more than it is governed by them, I commence with its diseases and affections.

The old régime labors at the relaxation of the ganglionic nerves and digestive canals in man, from his birth upwards, with such consequence, that we are almost tempted to hold it for refinement, because it is difficult to believe in the honesty of such immoderate blunders.

Directly upon entrance into the world, the unlucky sucklings are favored by their nurses with draughts from the camomile tea-pot, and consequently, all nurseries ring with the cries of stomach-ache. At the same time, both before and after weaning, they are fed with cows' milk *boiled.* Will not the doctors and nurses soon fall upon the bright idea of first milking the mother, and boiling her milk? They are fed with warm, even hot soup, and in order to crown the work of stomach destruction; they are dosed with medicine, as soon as the organism begins a remedial struggle against so many perversities, as soon as a primary symptom of disease appears.

Take young lions into such a régime, and you will soon see a race of lions with cramps and gripes in the bowels.

Not only human reason and human instinct, but the most recent experience gives the incontestable certainty, that children, in a diet of cool or cold food, without soups, of unboiled milk, and cold water, as the only drinks, *never* suffer from sickness of stomach, *never* have pains or gripes in the bowels, *never* have worms. If such children, through mistake, partake of unwholesome or poisonous things, they relieve themselves of them by energetic vomiting and diarrhœas, well observed, if nature be allowed to have its course, and its instinct be aided with cold water; but especially spared from swallowing medicines.

On the other hand, those unhappy martyrs of the old poisoning and effeminating system, pass through a childhood replete with suffering, and have before them the prospect of a life without health. When, by the said triple alliance of stomach-destroyers, the energy and activity of this important organ are impaired; then any slight inadvertence in diet, any overstepping of the bounds prescribed by the delicateness of constitution, brings on a disorder of the stomach, which cannot be removed otherwise than by abnormal exertion. Only eat somewhat over the usual quantity, or something difficult of digestion, and the stomach is not capable of doing its work of digestion; but it remains there till it has passed into putridity, and then the stomach must have recourse to some unusual help—to primary disease. Vomitings or diarrhœas come to the assistance. Instead of promoting this wholesome process with water, it is suppressed by medicine, and as soon as this has taken place, the organism must allow those morbid matters, which it was endeavoring to expel, to be firmly settled in itself by enveloping them in mucus and allowing them to indurate. Thus, then, the foundation is laid to the chronic misery that follows.

Children, in general, are remarkable for their health of stomach, which far exceeds the general average of persons advanced in years—and very naturally, because medicinal poisoning operates slowly and takes effect after a considerable interval. Most people think, however, that it lies in their nature; that the child's stomach can endure more than the adult's. We often hear it said, "such a youngster can eat anything!" Much rather say, "such a man can," because every grown creature has, from nature, stronger organs than the young undeveloped.

VI.

CURE OF THE PRIMARY DISEASES OF THE DIGESTIVE ORGANS IN GENERAL.

All these diseases are cured with the greatest certainty and promptness by water. The aim of all these cures, the inflammations in the bowels, also, not excepted, is the dissolution, and then the expulsion of morbific matters through vomiting and evacuations. There is no possibility of a real cure without these final results; if the acute struggle ceases without these results, it is certain that the irritating matters are fixed chronically in the stomach and bowels.

It is very evident in what manner water cures all these diseases. It is the only fluid capable of dissolving the viscous, slimy, morbid matters; secondly, by means of its coldness and decomposing power, it calls forth the elevated activity of the organs in question; and thirdly, it imparts to the stomach and bowels the fulness, which is necessary to evacuation.

(Of the effect and operation of the medical purgative remedies see farther on.)

The treatment in all these diseases consists in drinking, bandages, clysters, and sitz baths.

The measure of the drinking, the number of the clysters and sitz baths vary according to the variety and degree of the diseases, as also according to the constitutions of the patients. Generally, the instinct indicates the measure of the drinking, and of the clystering; the water-physician must determine the number and length of the sitz baths, if the patient does not possess the requisite hydriatic knowledge.

These diseases are all cured so surely and quickly by water, that the one so treated may soon go about his concerns again free from all after-pains.

VII.

NAUSEA AND VOMITING. DIARRHŒA.

Nauseousness may arise from ill-temper and imagination, from ossification and ulceration of the digestive organs, and particularly of the nerves of the same; such kind of nausea belongs to the secondary or destroying diseases.

Here we are speaking only of primary nausea, which is caused by nauseating matters in the stomach. These nauseating substances may be of various kinds, as was explained in the chapter on poisons. If poison, in the broader or stricter sense, be taken into a strong stomach, and water, or milk, or any mild and solvent fluid be drunk, there will always ensue thereupon nausea and vomiting, from the exertion of the organism to free itself of the nauseating substances. To vomit, it is necessary that the stomach possess a certain degree of muscular power, and, therefore, the quite weak and medicine-ruined stomach cannot, or only imperfectly, cleanse itself by vomiting. Vomiting arises from a violent contraction of the inferior parts of the stomach, thus raising its contents, and disgorging them upwardly.

The opinion often pronounced by the doctors, that difficult vomiting, after emetics, is a sign of strong stomach, is thoroughly false; it is a mark of a powerless stomach. The stronger the stomach, the more easily and energetically does it cast out of itself all poison-matters by vomiting, if its healing struggles be aided by water and milk. In the case of not violent poisons, of nauseating matters not properly of poisonous nature, water-drinking alone is sufficient to their radical expulsion through vomiting; with the stronger poisons, however, it is necessary to drink much unboiled sweet milk, so that the poison be enveloped and thereby retained in the milk, which then immediately curdles, cheese-like, in the stomach, and is prevented from exerting its corrosive power upon the coats of the same. This corroding power, if it is of a violent nature, so disables and cramps the stomach, that it cannot produce the curative vomiting at all, or at least not completely. Another sort of substances besides original poison, causes, likewise, primary vomiting, viz. when a stomach not without strength, has been overloaded with foods and drinks, especially with intoxicating drinks, hard of digestion, or mixed with poisons, and is unable to digest them, it endeavors, a few hours afterwards, to relieve itself of the same through vomiting, which is preceded by nauseousness. With such nauseating articles, water only, and not milk, must be drunk, for the purpose of exciting vomiting, because here nothing is necessary but the *mechanical* operations of the liquid to cleanse the stomach.

Every poisonous medicament, and every poison will produce vomiting with a strong and healthy stomach, if water and milk be drunk immediately after, and if quantity and quality are not of such degree that *instantaneous* death ensues.

When, however, nauseating matter is taken into the stomach, and is not removed through vomiting, because the necessary quantity of water and milk (or other mild liquid, as decoctions of harmless herbs in water, which, however, always operate less beneficially than water and milk) has not been drunk, then a vigorous, healthy, digestive organ unloads itself of these nauseous stuffs, at least partially, by means of diarrhœa, through the bowels.

Thus, when the nauseous substances have arrived at the ileum and jejunum (the absorbing intestines), the instinct of these organs is made aware, through disagreeable or corrosive affections, of the perniciousness of these substances, and absorbs, most probably, less of them than if they were wholesome and well-digested substances. The said bowels must, however, absorb much of them, and thus conduct it into the blood and entire body, because by reason of their construction and activity, they cannot arbitrarily desist from the peristaltic motion, and still less, close entirely the absorbent vessels. [The Constructor of the human organism, in placing an instinct in the human palate, has fully done his duty in regard to protection against poisons. If, despite his instinct, man still takes poison, it is an error which emanates from man's licentiousness (as vices do, also), and can in no wise be made a subject of complaint against the Creator.] These nauseous and poisonous stuffs that have now come through the small bowels into the evacuating bowels (large intestines), produce, in these latter intestines, tormenting and painful sensations ; the nauseous substances exercise their destroying power, and for this reason, the intestines endeavor to rid themselves as quickly as possible of them, which can be effected only by the secretion of much liquid. By means of the same, the intestines endeavor to wash themselves clean of the unwholesome matter, in which they are seldom completely successful without the assistance of water administered as injections. It is of itself evident, that the intestines are rendered uncommonly dry by the abnormal secretion of liquid and mucus, which is necessary to the production of the primary diarrhœa, and that the injection of water into the rectum is consequently an essential aid, and a support to the symptoms of reaction.

The primary diarrhœa following soon after eating unwholesome articles of food, lasts always but a short time. The critical diarrhœa, which arises in the water-cure, when morbid matters, which almost *always* are acrid medicaments, get released from old indurated mucus in the intestines, may continue for weeks and months, and still it is purely curative, health-restoring disease, and consequently by virtue of this character belongs to the acute diseases, to the chronic disease, however, by reason of its exceeding four weeks in duration. We see from this example, that the words acute and chronic are not suitable to our classification of diseases; it must, however, be observed, that the words "primary" and "secondary" in their true interpretation are likewise not so closely expressive, as the words "healing" and "destroying disease," and that we use them arbitrarily in a sense, which corresponds with our classification.

There is a destroying diarrhœa, which is no curative endeavor of the organism; which has its origin in the deepest ruin of the absorbent intestines, and carries with itself consumption. The chief distinctive mark between this secondary and the just mentioned primary diarrhœa consists herein, that the primary diarrhœa is frequently attended with a burning, and a feeling of great dryness in the anus (produced by the evacuated acrid matter), while on the contrary in the destroying diarrhœa this feeling is entirely wanting.

Between the two kinds of diarrhœa, that have just been considered, apparently holding the middle station, but in reality belonging to the primary class, is that diarrhœa, which is caused by a sudden and entire change in the food. The digestive juice always assumes that quality, which is most suited to the digestion of those foods generally eaten; is another sort of food suddenly eaten, which requires another quality of gastric juice, the unaccustomed foods are not at first easily and perfectly digested, and the stomach only adapts itself gradually to that state, which produces the suitable kind of digestive matter. During this period of transition the body clears itself by means of diarrhœas, of that portion of the unaccustomed food, which is not digested, and has frequently passed into putridity. Such a kind of diarrhœa needs the least of all a positive treatment, but in general requires simply non-interference and the guarantee of an undisturbed course of action, and quite especially no drugging. Water drinking according to the thirst, and one or two clysters daily is all the treatment necessary.

Such diarrhœas, arising from the strangeness of new aliments occur, for instance, in the too sudden weanings of sucking infants; more frequently in emigrations to a foreign zone, and most particularly in emigrations from cold climates to warmer and hot, where all the products have another nature than in the North; which diversity extends even to the productions of the same varieties.

VIII.

MUCOUS ENVELOPMENT OF MATTERS OF DISEASE, PARTICULARLY OF THE POISONOUS.

When poisonous and indigestible substances are not expelled by vomiting or diarrhœa in the manner just described, they must either remain in the alimentary canals, or be carried into the blood, and through the circulation of the same into the remotest parts of the whole body.

The manner in which the organism protects itself for a length of time against poisonous substances, which it cannot expel and which it is obliged to retain within itself, in order that they may not by their corroding power effect immediate destruction of the parts to which they have penetrated, appears at first view totally inexplicable.

The organism, which cannot through vomiting and diarrhœa rid itself of poisonous matter, which is lodged in it, conducts it over into the blood, and removes it in this manner from the digestive canals, *if the digestive organs are possessed of the requisite strength for so doing. When they have lost this power, the poisonous and morbific matters remain in them, and fix themselves in indurated mucus on to the walls of the stomach and of the bowels.*

We will first take into consideration the question, how the organism manages with poisonous and medicinal substances, when they are carried by the circulation of the blood into the innermost parts of the body, and it has not the strength and the means to enable it to free itself of the same through boils and eruptions, of which we shall speak farther on.

How is it possible, that the body can harbor in itself acrid poisons for a long time with apparent health? How is it, that the poisons, while lying in the flesh and bone, do not corrode in like manner, as, when driven by water-cure out upon the surface, they do the skin in boils, and even eat through the linen compresses?

The anatomical knife gives us no information on this head, because the matters of disease—whether medicinal poisons, or acrid humors, from sharp high seasoned foods, or stagnated and refuse particles of the body—are divided into such minute atoms, that the eye does not recognise any what of them.

Just as little may we expect enlightenment from the

old pathology, which gives information of nothing else than of its own incompetency and inconsistency. When one cons over the pages of the allopathic pathologies, he meets in the case of almost every disease with the edifying information: "of the causes and manner of origination of this disease, the greatest pathologists and physiologists are of different and mostly contradictory opinion." Very edifying; for where error is, there always are disagreements and contradictions, in truth is alone unity and agreement.

Still, despite the contradictions of the most renowned pathologists, we can, with such decided certainty, find the solution of this problem through combination, that it can be doubted by no one, except those whom interest urges thereto.

What does the human body do when large, visible, inimical substances are driven into it through external force? What, for instance, with the leaden bullet? Its first endeavor is to throw off the foreign mass by suppuration; when this is impossible, or it is forced from its purpose by plasters and medicine, *it conducts to the spot a great quantity of mild mucus-like humor, envelopes it therein, and forms around it a net-work wherein it holds captive the bullet and the poisonous effect of the lead.* The organism endeavors this same procedure, with the minute poisonous and inimical substances, which have been forced upon it through the digestion—if it is obstructed in its endeavors to expel them again by acute force.

This theory is founded upon the incontrovertible principle of nature in the elementary and organic world, that nature operates similarly under similar circumstances. Hence, the theory produced loses none of its certainty, because we are not able to recognise with the unaided eye, on account of their minuteness, the inimical atoms and the minute net-work around them, and to exhibit them by section.

Many bodies exist without our being able to see them. The mites, which cause the itch, have but recently become perceptible to the eye by artificial optical assistance; the minute animalculæ, in infusions and in water, have long been unknown, and now magnified by the hydro-oxygen microscope, these formerly invisible pigmies are enlarged to the size of a crocodile or an elephant. It is highly probable that at a future time some one will succeed in laying open to the eye the matters of disease in dissected bodies, as that the atoms of the same shall be made apparent. The whole of these matters collectively, exert, even now, a general effect upon the observant eye, through the abnormal color, which they impart to the flesh of the patient that has died of chronic disease. When these foreign matters have a marked color, first, the mucus, and second, the flesh, partakes somewhat of it. If, however, this color is not very striking (as is generally the case), then the flesh must have a pale non-normal tincture, from the whitish color of the mucus. The fact has been actually ascertained from butchers, that the flesh of such animals as, notwithstanding good feeding, will not fatten (which can only proceed from chronic sickness), generally has an unnatural, pale, whitish color.

The difference of the internal flesh color in healthy and chronically-diseased persons, would show itself still more characteristically distinct, if bodies of both kinds slain on the battle-field, should be examined.

The flesh of animals has always the same blood color, because in the green republics of the woods there can be no chronic sickness, since there are there no doctors, no apothecaries, and no distilleries of intoxicating liquors.

Now, we will consider the second question of this chapter, namely, the fixture of poisonous medicinal substances in the digestive canals themselves.

A strong digestive organ will rid itself, as we have seen, in some manner, of the medicinal substances forced upon it. When, however, the use of medicine is perseveringly adhered to for a length of time, the walls of the stomach and bowels become gradually desiccated by the constant secretion of mucus, to which alternative the digestive canals are driven, in order to protect themselves against the sharp and corrosive medicaments, and thus, in places, the corrosive power of the medicaments effects a ruination of the mucous glands and of the nerves. Now, on these most exhausted and ruined places, the mucous accumulations with which the poisons are mixed, become fixed, and harden, by degrees, to that stone-like concretion which is commonly called tartar. The tartar, which, with persons of foul stomach, settles upon the teeth, is likewise nothing else than indurated mucus. The more now, the use of medicine is persevered in, the more the mucus generated is mixed with the medicine, and adheres along with it firmly to the walls of the stomach and bowels. In such a way, many persons carry about with them in their digestive canals a small apothecary shop. It is evident, that the medicaments firmly encased in mucus and tartar, inasmuch as no dissolving power, neither air nor water can reach them, must continue to retain their peculiar strength and peculiar taste, until they are again subjected to the decomposing power of the elements, which in the lifetime of the patient is only practicable by a water-cure. If the water does not dissolve this indurated mucus, then the solution and decomposition of the medicaments therein contained, do not take place until after the death and decomposition of the patient through the decomposing power of the elements.

It is a circumstance well known to physicians, that in very weak digestive canals, medicaments may lie undigested; I remember, that long before the water-cure became known, my physician at that time, Dr. H., in C., while I had an intermitting fever, would give me no china in substantial form, because, in my too weak stomach, "it might remain undigested as a crudity in my stomach." That appeared to me, at the time, impossible. I questioned physicians as to the possibility of it, and received affirmative answer; I searched in medical works, and found it confirmed. If, now, many physicians still deny these facts and the possibility of the same, I am in no manner surprised, because, in the present struggle between medicine and water-cure, a mass of untruths is set forth to the people by the physicians concerning both systems, contrary to their better knowledge, in order to dispute the results of the water-cure and to vindicate medicine.

I have shown that the fixture of medicaments in indurated mucus finds its fullest explanation in the laws of physiology. The contrary would be a contradiction to physiology; it is an utter impossibility that weakened bowels, which have long been allopathically fed with acrid and poisonous medicaments, can constantly retain the power of expelling the poisons along with the mucus which they generate. Many persons may suppose that the potions afterwards taken must again dissolve the mucus, and that it cannot, therefore, continue fixed for lifetime. To that I reply the following:

First, Knowledge, established by experience, teaches the contrary: viz. in dissections it is not seldom that tartar is found in the digestive canals, which requires a long time for its formation; over which, consequently, many fluids have passed without dissolving it.

Second, Of all drinks water alone possesses this dissolvent power, and then only when somewhat more of it is drunk than the thirst requires. For what the thirst demands is quickly absorbed, and accordingly has no time to dissolve a tough, still less a stone-like, concretion.

Third, The digestive canals retain, for the purposes of solution, that water drunk beyond the thirst, so long as it is needed for the solution, if they have the strength to expel the dissolved mucus, together with the poison contained therein. If they do not possess this strength, then the solution would be a misfortune, and consequently, the digestive organs empty themselves quickly of the superfluous water, and allow of no solution, in consequence of the instinct, which is placed not only in the palate, but also in all the organs.

Hence it follows, that the solution of the indurated and stone-like mucus is only practicable through the agency of water, and by water treatment; and that without this the mucus must remain in the body till death in the form of tartar.

Not all medicaments have this effect of hardening the mucus, and coating the digestive canals with tartar, but in the same degree more or less, according as they are stronger or weaker poisons, and more or less administered for a length of time. One may always reckon with certainty upon indurated mucus in patients that have taken much of medicinal purgative remedies, and much of constipating remedies, because they dry up the digestive canals in an extraordinary manner. Laudanum in particular is disposed to take up its abode and remain in the bowels.

It is of itself evident, that those parts of the stomach and bowels, to which the tartar adheres, must soon organically perish, and pass into induration and cartilage. However, we return again hereafter to this subject.

In the foregoing has been shown, that the medicaments must retain their peculiar power and peculiar taste in the mucous indurations, until the mucus is dissolved, and the poisonous matters become exposed to the elements. Therefore, in the statement, that in the water cure patients have, during a vomiting crisis, vomited out medicinal stuffs, which they had taken several years before; and in the statement, that these substances had retained their own peculiar taste, and oftentimes perceptibly their own color, there is contained nothing, which offers the slightest contradiction to the laws of physiology; and the laughter, which some physicians make use of against such statements, springs either from gross ignorance or from conscious untruth.

The weaker the stomach, the more unaltered remain the taste and strength of the medicaments enveloped in mucus. If the stomach, however, is somewhat stronger, it attempts at least through its own peculiar juice a relative alteration of the administered poisonous drugs, before it resigns itself to the necessity of retaining in itself the poisons together with the mucus. When a patient in the water cure gets a vomiting crisis, and in the ejected morbid matter can plainly taste a medicine that was taken some time ago, then he may rest assured that this crisis will continue some time, and will not cease until the ejected matter loses its marked medicinal taste. That, which in such a crisis is first discharged, is naturally the poison that was last taken, and the last discharged is that first taken, and first settled in the stomach. At first, however, the stomach has still strength to make a relative change in the poisons, the very powerful ones excepted; which change indeed never reaches actual digestion, which however somewhat diminishes the strength of the poison, and thus divests it of its peculiar taste, so that it is converted into a more or less acrid, but always an undigested and poisonous, crudity.

The theme of sliming or mucous envelopment is one of the most important in the doctrine of disease. The real genuine sliming by abnormal secretions from the everywhere extended mucous glands can never be produced but by sharp poisons, which very seldom come from other hands than those of the drug-physician, and the so-called slime-dissolving remedies of the doctors are in reality slime-generating remedies.

When it is said of foods and drinks, that they cause a flow of mucus, it is not the real true mucus, i. e. mucus generated and secreted from the mucous glands, but rather a transition of the chyle into a mucus-like substance from want of strength, especially from want of decomposing power in the weak digestive organs, which always has its cause in poisons and insufficient use of water.

Of the so-called slime-dissolving and purging remedies of the doctors, we shall speak more at large hereafter.

I cannot conclude this so exceedingly important theme of sliming, before I overthrow still an argument of the doctors, wherein they deny the permanent continuance of the matters of disease in the body.

From the nature of poisons we have seen, that, when they are introduced into the stomach and not expelled again through vomiting, they either adhere to the walls of the digestive canals in hardened mucus or slime, or are taken up by the digestive organs and carried into the blood. These are carried by the blood and circulation thereof into all the various and innermost parts of the body and there deposited with the other constituents of the blood to afford nourishment to the same, and to renew the constant wear and tear of the body.

When many physicians, for the purpose of disputing the water-cure, deny this now, they contradict not only the very physiological laws which are proclaimed from their lecturing desks, but they deny all efficaciousness to their own medicaments. *If the medicaments did not pass into the blood, and through it into the body, they could have no effect farther than, at most, upon the digestive organs, into which always they make their way.*

Supposing the medicinal and poisonous substances passed into the blood, but not in their medicinal quality, but entirely divested of their poison, completely digested, made like to the blood, which is prepared from the usual aliments ; *then again they could possess no medicinal efficaciousness, and in general no other power than that which is possessed by every natural, and, as pointed out by instinct, agreeable food.*

Thus the physicians, when they pretend that their poisons and medicaments are capable of being assimilated, not only contradict physiological laws but themselves also, in the most direct manner, inasmuch as in all diseases which have their seat otherwise than in the digestive canals, they thereby deny that medicinal effect, which, however, at every other opportunity they avow, and upon which their whole doctrine of cure is founded.

The more clever ones among the physicians have very well comprehended this double contradiction, and they admit that the drugs retaining their medicinal quality are carried by the circulation of the blood into all parts of the body, but usually maintain that the medicinal and poisonous substances are again promptly thrown off by the evaporations from the skin.

This fundamentally false doctrine I must yet disprove, before I can conclude this chapter.

The blood is impelled into all, even into the innermost solid parts, as, for instance, into the bones through the circulation, which is driven by means of the immense muscular power of the heart, so that the substance which, being worn out, has passed off, is again replaced anew by the blood. So long as poisonous and medicinal substances are still to be found in the blood of the large veins, they cannot exert any, or but slight injurious effects, because they are not mixed with the healthy parts of the blood, because in the blood itself there are no nerves, and because they are rapidly hurried through the veins. As soon, however, as the blood has arrived at the place of its destination, through the innumerable small veins, it is decomposed more or less by the organic power into its constituent parts, and out of the various constituent parts are formed the various juices and substances which it stands in need of for its nutrition: the hairy matter, muscular matter, the nervous matter, the seminal matter, marrow, &c., &c. Into all these solid, and also into all fluid substances, now the very minute and consequently very numerous particles of poison pass, which have entered into the circulation, and are through the same carried into all parts of the body. As soon as the particles of poison are in this manner separated from the blood, and have settled in the solid and organically vital parts of the body (the blood is not as yet an organically developed body, but the material for the organic formations of the human body), they begin to exercise their annihilating power, which is, however, kept down by the organism for a length of time, by secreting from the everywhere existing mucous glands and glandules mild mucous humors, and therewith enveloping the particles of poison. The labor of generation of, and envelopment in mucus, is infinitely easier and requires infinitely less strength, than the work of elimination of the poison through the organ of the skin.

When the body is poisoned with drugs, this elimination through the skin can never take place readily, and never without the help of water. Their elimination cannot take place readily, because those parts of the body into which the particles of poison arrive, together with the rest of the particles of blood to nourish, to replace the worn out and refuse substance, are not organically inclined to secrete immediately again those newly arrived substances, because the secretions from organically vivified parts of the body ensue, according to normal manner, not till a long time afterwards; and not till such time, as these substances being worn out and exhausted have become refuse. Those substances, which have to-day been deposited in organic parts of the body, will, in normal manner, be excreted again the last of all substances which to-day are in the body. The older is always excreted before the fresher and newer. *Thus the assertion, that the medicinal poisons are quickly discharged again out of the body, is a contradiction against the laws of physiology, and consequently a decided untruth.*

Without help of water the complete expulsion of poisonous substances through the organ of the skin is never possible, not even slowly, if this poisoning has been carried to such an extent, as it usually is with most of the allopathic treatments.

To excrete poisonous matters from the skin requires, however, still more strength of the skin, than to excrete the refuse matters of assimilation, and therefore the former is still less possible without the help of water. By far the greater number of powerful poisons, when conducted from the internal organs to the skin, excite boils and eruptions, which cause a violent burning and stinging in the skin. Even the first appearance of these critical poison-discharging exanthems is very seldom out of the water-cure, and then only with persons of very strong constitutions. But the maintenance of these exanthems until the body is thoroughly cleansed is not possible with the strongest persons without water treatment, because the skin system becomes gradually dried out by such secretions, and in places at least disorganized, if the acridities of the secretions are not mildened by dilutions with water, and if the skin is not bathed with and allowed to absorb much water, to replace the elastic fluid, which it must produce in abnormal quantity to carry off the poisonous matters.

The less violent poisons may in many persons, especially those of very fat and coarse system of skin, be discharged without any exanthems, but likewise not without water. The burning and itching, which such critical transpirations and transudations irritate in the skin, must likewise be cooled by water, if the acrid matters, which cause these sensations, are not gradually to desiccate the skin, and thus make it wholly incapable of the abnormal activity required to throw off the poison.

Farthermore, the necessary cleansing of the pores and keeping them open during such like critical transudations and exanthems can only be attained by frequent moistening of the skin with water.

Finally, the skin can receive from water only the ab normal supply of oxygen and hydrogen, which as before shown must attend every abnormal activity of the body.

In all these demonstrations of the impossibility of the excretion of poison without help of water, regard only has been had to the cutaneous system, and it has been shown, that complete elimination is even then not possible, when the poisonous substances have arrived at the skin.

Hereafter I will show, that it is not possible for these poisonous drugs and spices to be expedited from the innermost parts of the body to the skin without the help of water.

IX.

THE NATURE AND PURPOSE OF FEVER.

Infinite time and pains have been expended in the investigation of the nature and the causes of fever by the thousands, who have in this century devoted their whole lives professionally to the curing of diseases. But alas the riddle remained unsolved, despite so many guessers and counsellors.

Hahnemann is of the opinion, that perhaps it will never be granted to humanity to fathom, to determine the inward nature of fever and of the chronic diseases. If, however, some one should succeed in so doing, the explanation would be so simple, so evident, so disrobed of learned subtility, that it would captivate every human understanding, and fill it with a new flood of light. This is most certainly true!

Fever is—but, man, what art thou attempting? What science in two centuries has been unable to solve—whereon Boerhave and his consorts of glory have ground to dulness their wisdom teeth—that secret wilt thou break open and unriddle? Well, I draw the curtains of modesty over my face, with maiden bashfulness I cast down mine eyes, with blushes on my cheeks I beg consideration for my learned stupidity, and stammer as follows: *Fever is nothing more and nothing less than the effect of any and every violent exertion, which exceeds the normal and conservative powers of the body.*

Run hard, or have a bad wound on your body to heal, or beget a human being, or bear a child, and you thence get a fever just as perfect, but not of so long duration, as when the body reacts violently against a suppressed perspiration, or in general is striving to drive morbific matters from the internal parts to the skin.

There are only three characteristic marks of fever which are brought on by every violent exertion, viz. heat of the body, rapid pulse, and dry tongue, which by longer duration of the exertion becomes a parching thirst. All other symptoms of a fever of disease, are not symptoms of fever, but effects of those matters of disease, which are to be expurged by means of the fever. For this reason these other symptoms are just as changing and various as the nature of the morbific matters, or as the organs are different upon which the matters have thrown themselves. Are these matters, through obstructed perspiration, settled particularly in the head, then arises an inflammation of the brain; if upon the lungs, then, an inflammation of the lungs; and a nervous, or typhus fever, if upon the nerves.

The physicians, indeed, premise still more necessary marks of fever, viz. the chill before the heat, also depression of the general strength of the organism, and finally, destruction of the functions of digestion and evacuation. But firstly, the chill is not the fever, but the preparation to the fever; the start, as it were, before the fever. Secondly, the depression of the organism results less from the fever than from the disease, against which the fever is a token of reaction; and this depression is, in the water-treatment, far less sensible than in the medical; is, therefore, a partial effect of the medicaments. Instances are known to me wherein persons with fever have, under the water-cure, walked upwards of three miles to get to the bath in the open air, and, indeed, in raw weather with the best consequences. Thirdly, the destruction of digestive energies takes place always in every case under medical treatment, but very frequently not at all under the hydriatic, and always for a short time only. It is nothing rare in critical feverish conditions in the water-cure, that during the same the patient eats with better appetite, digests and evacuates better than many persons in the old régime during their healthy days. Consequently, the disturbance of the digestive energies is by no means a necessary effect of the fever, but of the medical treatment of the same.

In all these violent diseases it would scarcely require to be proved that the causes of these diseases are foreign material substances in the body, if the so-called science had not so automatonized the people, that they believe more readily the puppet in the professorial chair, than the innermost infallible human perceptions. Does it not, in all these diseases, lie perceptibly in and upon the diseased organ? does it not sting, and burn, and press? In inflammation of the chest, what compressed anguish, and what stitches, like with glowing daggers, as if an Etna lay upon the lungs, and his fires were raging therein! Here it sits! oh! here it pierces, here it burns, here it cramps! oh! oh! cries the poor patient. "But, nay," says the wooden science, "you err grossly, it is not foreign matters that afflict you, it is rather ——." Yes, there the breath of the discourse ceases, there it stagnates. The wisest and most celebrated among physicians have honestly confessed that they know nothing of the internal nature and process of diseases. But the narrow-minded content themselves with high-sounding phrases, void of sense and purport, as they twang from the lecturer's chair, and with faithful devotion they learn the stupidity by heart, and pay themselves and their like with the false coin, which weighs nothing, but only jingles.

In common life, we are accustomed to call fever that condition of body which is produced by abnormal physiological activity of the inner man without external and arbitrary effort. We will take the word fever here without farther argument, in the ordinary sense of fever of disease, i. e. fever accompanied by symptoms of disease.

In all abnormal efforts of the organism, there is more oxygen and hydrogen gas consumed than in the normal condition. In order to draw more oxygen from the air the lungs respire more rapidly than ordinarily, which produces an acceleration in the throb of the heart and pulse; from this accelerated circulation of the blood arises the fever heat. The fever-thirst arises very naturally from the abnormally great consumption of oxygen and hydrogen. These two gases are, as was before shown, the fundamental conditions of all assimilation and secretion, since the solid can be transformed into fluid only through the agency of hydrogen, and the fluid into solid only through the agency of oxygen, gas.

In this manner the nature of fever is very simply and clearly comprehended. The causes and purpose of fever will be given farther on. Let any one compare my explanation of fever with those before given, and he will perceive that mine alone has claim to the predicates of simplicity and clearness. I have also had the satisfaction to perceive that a number of authors have borrowed from me, and consequently approved of the declaration of the nature of fever given by me, before me entirely unknown. If, in so doing, they have not named myself as the originator of it, and have, in part, assumed to themselves the title of authorship, it is only an occurrence that has in similar cases been repeated a thousand times, and must necessarily proceed from the vanity of contracted souls. In the majority of hydriatic works by mediciners and non-mediciners, that have appeared since the publication of my miscellanies, my explanation of fever has been adopted.

X.

THE INTERNAL PROCESS OF TAKING COLD.

Colds play a principal part in the pathology of the mediciners, as well as of the laymen. Concerning the internal processes of those diseases arising from colds, we have had heretofore not so much incorrect ideas as much rather no ideas at all; these processes have been developed first in my doctrine of disease.

If a human body is quite free from morbific humors (foreign matters more or less poisonous), then taking cold could have a morbid effect only, if the nerves were extremely weak and diseased, and this disease could consist only in nervous irritations, depressions, and cramps. But in a body free from foreign humors, there are no diseased nerves, and consequently, sickness can never arise in such manner from colds, if there are no foreign humors in the body.

The skin can perform its necessary business of excretion only when its pores are open and it is warm. These two conditions cannot be permanently maintained but by means of cold water. Indeed, warmth can be maintained around the body for a length of time by confining the immediate atmosphere of the skin with thick coverings of imperfect conductors of heat; but such a manner of maintaining the warmth of the skin has two decided disadvantages; first, that the skin, which not only exhales the insensible perspiration, but must also absorb from the atmosphere, can then induct into the body only corrupt atmospheric nutrition (see under air baths), and second, by this artificial retention of the transpired warmth, the power of the skin to generate warmth becomes gradually weaker, and consequently, more and more covering becomes necessary.

Because in the old régime the skin cannot generate of itself the warmth necessary to transpiration, it becomes obstructed so soon as the accustomed artificial aids are not satisfactorily guaranteed. This obstruction of transpiration is the so-called catarrh or cold which, however, as before said, can only produce disease when morbific humors (i. e. matters that are or have become foreign, and are not exhaled in time from the body) are present in the body.

When under such circumstances the transpiration stagnates for a length of time by reason of insufficient warmth of skin, the matters to be transpired take an abnormal course towards the inward parts of the body, or at least the fluid matter, that should have evaporated, remains an abnormal length of time within the body, *and dissolves by reason of its fluidity many of those mucous particles in which the foreign, and especially the poisonous matters, lay enveloped.* It must, then, necessarily result, that these morbid humors which have been thus freed from their mucous envelopment, produce by their acrid and corrosive properties pains in those parts of the body with which they come in contact. The organism can operate in two ways with these free humors, viz. it can either endeavor to conduct them to the skin, and there excrete them, or it can envelope them again with newly-generated mucus. The first is a struggle for radical cure, and is undertaken by the organism the more decidedly and powerfully, according as it is stronger and healthier. The second course is a shift, which the ruined organism adopts, and to which even a sound organism is forced, when its endeavor to cure itself is suppressed through medicinal treatment, i. e. either through blood-letting or poisoning.

A necessary consequence of the elucidation just given by me is the conclusion that under preparatory treatment of catarrhal complaints with water, the act of taking cold, i. e. the setting free of the foreign humors from their mucous envelopment by means of the fluids that should have been transpired, remaining an abnormal length of time in the body, can become a means of cure in the truest sense of the word, a means of the radical expulsion of the morbid humors. The conclusion is most substantially correct, when there is previous strength of the skin and of the general organism sufficient for going victoriously through the struggle, and when there has been previous water-treatment.

The originator of the systematic water-cure, uses, for the purpose of intentional catarrhs and colds, or the dissolving of the old mucus by obstructions of the exhalations, those half baths, which I have called "fever-producing baths."

These half-baths are employed to change atonic conditions of disease (i. e. conditions of disease without pain, and devoid of any symptoms of reaction) into tonic. They must not be employed if the nerves are considerably affected, or if the cutaneous system is inactive. In general none but the perfect master of the water-cure system should meddle with them.

The stronger the organism is at the time of its infection with matters of disease, so much the sooner ensues an acute disease after taking cold; so much the purer and more marked also does the disease resulting from cold partake of the inflammatory character, and so much the freer is it of nervous symptoms.

With very vigorous persons the inflammatory affection ensues always within a few days after the cold, and just as soon, and still sooner, follows the crisis in the water-cure, sometimes immediately after the fever-generating half-bath.

But the unfortunate beings who have a shattered nervous system, never get inflammatory affections after a cold, because it requires good, or tolerably good, nerves to produce them; those unfortunates suffer the most after colds from increased nervous afflictions, less from rheumatic pains, and not at all from the inflammatory. An organism with shattered nerves can do nothing but immediately re-envelope with mucus those morbific humors, which are set free. This exertion, however, of itself so trivial, produces, in combination with the constringent prime effect of the cold upon the nerves, an increase of the nervous sufferings. Hence it follows, that persons with shattered nerves must, under all circumstances, carefully guard against taking cold, and this also while under the water-treatment, until such time that the nerves have gained strength and healthiness therefrom.

From the above-shown difference in the effects of a cold upon healthy and diseased nerves it is argued, that that method of cure which changes the rheumatic and inflammatory disposition of disease gradually into a nervous, is by all means thoroughly false and ruinous; and that that method which produces the contrary change, must decidedly be the true method. Thousands and millions of times has medicine effected that disastrous change, and never has it produced a single instance of the last-named change, which leads to a true cure. Only water, only nature's medical art has the power to work out such a victorious change, which then is always the transition to the most complete cure.

Every person, who does not pursue internal and external water diet, does not transpire readily enough the refuse-grown substance, has therefore diseased matters in his body, and can, by taking cold, bring upon himself a disease. No wild beast, no wild man can be morbidly affected from the most violent cold, i. e. from transpirations for a long time entirely suppressed, because no old foreign substances are present in the body. If the external cold reaches such an unusual degree, that the organism cannot react against it, then it is possible that such a healthy being may, through withdrawal of all warmth, grow numb and perish, but never can any sickness follow from restoration of warmth.

To attain to such enviable ruggedness and incapability of taking cold, it is not necessary that we become wild; much rather, we may remain perfectly tame and comfortable, and be just as healthy as the tiger or polar bear—if we return to first principles, to the water-cure and water-diet. Such health will be guaranteed to the new-born babe, if it is reared in the water-diet; with him, however, who has grown up under the old régime, the diet is of little avail before he has been born anew by a course of water-treatment.

If any one is disposed to learn whether he is entirely free of foreign humors, is absolutely healthy, he can best make the test by intentionally contracting a severe cold. However, this may only be allowable when a water-physician is at hand to prevent any evil consequences, and when the state of the experimenter approaches nearly to that of health, which, in common life, is entitled extraordinarily healthy.

With a vigorous organism, which has for a considerable length of time pursued the water-diet (without being perfectly pure, however), a strong critical perspiration will break out, probably the next night after the contraction of the cold, and thus the matter is ended. With a healthy person under the usual diet, an acute disease will ensue, and, under water-treatment, disappear in a few days, without leaving a vestige behind.

The chronic patient should guard himself carefully against contracting any cold, because he can no longer produce any healing disease.

There are, certainly, very few persons in Europe that can bid defiance to any cold. These few would, in the Graefenberg water-cure, get no kind of crisis whatever. All others would do well to take in hand the water-purification of their bodies, which is attained so much the sooner the healthier their organism is. Very vigorous persons get, in the Graefenberg water-cure, eruptions within the first few days, while the weak and enfeebled require weeks and months.

XI.

DRINKING OF COLD WATER WHEN HEATED.

The cooling of the body internally through cold-water drinking while, or after being heated, operates in like manner as the cooling of the skin by ablutions, always refreshing and agreeable, and never produces sickness nor malady in a *healthy* person. Are we, indeed, to believe that nature has implanted in her creatures this ardent desire after cold water, if to appease it were injurious? Oh, the all-loving, noble Nature has given to man, as also to the beasts, no propensity the appeasing of which renders him unhappy or unhealthy! But cultivation, i. e. those distortions and distractions of civilization of which Europe is so proud, and which are continually approaching nearer and nearer to the absurdities of the Chinese—that has perverted most conditions and circumstances, and plunged them into misery and error!

Every beast, when it is heated, drinks with eagerness great quantities of cold water, and well it agrees with him. Only civilized man and the civilized horse are the sufferers thereby; for these poor creatures have a body always so full of corrupt matters, that any interrupted perspiration makes them sicken—thanks to the poisoning science! On the contrary, the wild horse, because it lives in the natural water-régime, is as healthy and as hardy as any other animal; even the horses of the Indians know of no trouble from this source, and, after being heated, drink with impunity, cold water, without being afterwards set in motion or receiving any covering.

If cold-drinking, when heated, were injurious, hey! Messrs. Doctors, what would have become of your ancestors in their wild hunting expeditions? From what medical bench was preached to the wild Germans, and to the savages of the present day, the precautions against cold water? And were and are these wild gentlemen of the woods perhaps pulmonary wheezers and asthmatics? And have you ever found a savage or a man of nature anywhere, who does not drink cold water when heated? In the moon perhaps, but not on earth.

Every one who is perfectly free of foreign matters, may drink cold water after the most intense over-heating of the body, and then at pleasure either heat himself still more, or allow himself to cool. Experience has already confirmed this.

But whoever has grown up in the régime of a false diet, and still more, whoever has swallowed the poisons of medicine, cannot drink in an over-heated state, if he does not continue in a state of activity, which will maintain the heat in him, unless he has previously purified himself completely by the water-treatment.

XII.

DYSENTERY.

REMARK.—When, in this work, the distinguishing symptoms of the different diseases are given under the title, "symptoms of the disease," these symptoms are always taken from those marks which characterize the disease, never from the nature of the disease, or from the causes of the disease, which two last subjects are treated immediately after the specification of the symptoms.

(1) *Symptoms of the Dysentery.*—Violent pains in the evacuating intestine (rectum), and sometimes in the other intestines also, attended with constant desire to evacuate and proportionately small stools. At first the evacuations consist only of the excrements in the bowels, but afterwards at a later and advanced stadium of the disease, which is chiefly the consequence of medicinal treatment, they consist mostly of greenish foul slime, which is passed only with great difficulty and straining. If blood is min-

gled with the evacuation, or preponderates in the mixture, it is called the bloody flux. When the false formations of inflammation arise through wrong treatment of the dysentery (of this see inflammatory diseases) cuticular and polypus-like formations are also evacuated. Farther, the dysentery passes under false treatment sometimes into ulceration of the bowels, more frequently into mortification, which then speedily produces death.

(2) *The Nature and Condition of Disease in Dysentery* is an inflammation in the large intestines, most frequently in the rectum, so that the excrements can with difficulty, or not at all, pass by the inflamed part, and hence arises the pressing desire to stool without the ability of effecting an evacuation. The causes of dysentery lie almost always in the corruption of the air, of the water, or of the food; colds and a previous predisposition to dysentery are co-operating causes. This latter consists chiefly in this, that in the coatings of the large intestines acrid or poisonous substances lie enveloped in mucus, which mucus is dissolved by the moisture repressed by the closing of the pores by cold; whereupon, then, in co-operation with the above-mentioned corruption of the elements or of the aliments, more morbid matters are accumulated in the bowels, against which the organism reacts with an inflammation, and thus endeavors to effect its cure.

Moreover, I must confess that I have not as yet succeeded in investigating the processes so clearly and thoroughly of the epidemic diseases as I have the processes of the non-epidemic.

(3) *The operation and effect of the water-treatment on the Dysentery.*

Remark.—In representing the effects of water on the

various diseases, I have always in view the true hydriatic treatment, according to the method of Vincent Priessnitz.

The water which is drunk always passes with great rapidity, and in inflammatory diseases, with uncommon rapidity through the whole circulation of the blood, and arrives very soon through the small veins of the bowels at the inflamed parts thereof; it dilutes and weakens the acrid humors, and thus renders them milder, and by means of its fluidity promotes their expulsion through the various excretory functions. The water taken as drink does not reach as such the cavities of the large intestines, since it is previously absorbed in the small ones; but, for the speedy cure of the dysentery, as of every inflammation, the application of a great quantity of water in its original substance is highly salutary; therefore, in the dysentery, a great many water clysters must be given, which come directly to the inflamed part of the bowels, where the proper seat of the disease lies. The water cools the inflammation, dilutes and qualifies the acrid morbid matters, which, through the reaction, are secreted partly from the internal parts of walls of the bowels, and discharged into the hollow spaces of the intestines, and which, for the rest part, have come into the canal of the large intestines through unwholesome foods and the corruption of the elements. Farthermore, the water gives to the bowels the necessary fulness, which facilitates evacuation, and in such manner washes them clear of all morbific humors. The water finally supplies the oxygen and hydrogen, which, in all inflammations, is consumed in abnormal quantity, without which the false formations of inflammation arise. Sitz-baths and wet compresses around the abdomen, make the work of cure complete.

When the dysentery-patient is reduced by medical treatment to that condition in which the transpirations of the skin, together with the alvine evacuations, have become obstructed and stagnated, then the water must first in wet sheet envelopments be directed towards re-animating the activity of the skin, which it arouses through its afore-described effect upon the human organism. Also, when there is considerable fever preceding the inclination to stool, a short envelopment is necessary.

The operation of water in the dysentery is therefore the cleansing of the large bowels of the foreign matters, against which the organism struggles so violently, and thus the water-cure is an assistant to the reactive struggle.

(4) *The effects of the medical treatment* upon the dysentery are according to the variousness of the remedies applied, partly of moderate, partly of vast injury. To the moderately injurious belong the slimy and oily remedies, which sometimes are given alone, when the symptoms do not rise to great violence ; but these remedies can never effect a cure. The administered oil burdens the stomach exceedingly ; it does not pass directly through the bowels, but is, for the most part, absorbed in the small intestines, consequently but a small portion reaches that part of the bowels, where the inflammation and proper seat of the disease lies. Even then it is of very inconsiderable benefit, because no inflammation can be cooled with oil, but only with water, because the oil possesses no dissolving power, because it can by no means penetrate into the very delicate and minute spaces, and because it contains neither oxygen nor hydrogen, which, in every inflammation, are of the most cogent necessity if they are to issue salutarily.

That that part of the oil, which is absorbed in the small

intestines, and thus conducted into the blood, can likewise exercise no salutary effect upon the disease, is evident from analogous causes.

Frequently a vomitive is administered immediately at the commencement of the dysentery, and this is still more in accordance with the characteristic spirit of medicine; it is a poisonous coercive remedy, which withholds the organism from its curative endeavor, either obstructing this endeavor or utterly rendering it impossible, just according to the strength of the patient.

The opiate medicaments, which are so very frequently administered in dysentery, operate in like manner. Their poisonous effects cripple the organism; hence the symptoms of reaction must in consequence thereof grow weaker, and on suitable repetition of the poisonings must finally cease, either because death, the grand colleague of the mediciners, gradually steps in, or because the organism desists from its struggle, and resorts to envelopment of the morbific matter in mucus. In this manner either death by mortification is incurred by the above-mentioned and other poisons, or chronic indurations and disorganizations form themselves in the inflamed parts, which are followed by tedious life-long complaints. This last we find noticed in all the medical pathologies, where indeed it is not at the same time mentioned, that the organic transformations and ravages are the effect of the poisonous suppression of the symptoms of reaction of the dysentery. But physiology affords proof to this, and moreover it has been confirmed a thousand times by experience. Never after hydriatic treatment has there arisen a chronic ailing in the evacuating bowel, and never has a patient under such treatment died of dysentery. I make here the explicit observation, that, when I speak of hydriatic treatment, I mean a treatment conducted from beginning to end with water, and exclude a previous medicinal one.

In the dysentery, as in every primary disease, the palate manifests a strong desire for cold water, and in every primary disease there must to a hair just so much be drunk as the thirst requires, and not a drop more.

XIII.

CHOLERA.

THERE is no fixed boundary to be drawn between the sporadic and Asiatic cholera, as in general nowhere between neighboring diseases can certain fixed boundaries be drawn.

(1) *Symptoms of the Cholera.*—Sometimes it is preceded by fore-tokens, frequently not.

The fore-tokens are dejectedness of mind and anxiety, weariness of the limbs and dizziness, in connexion with disturbances in the digestive functions, especially with diarrhœa.

The symptoms of cholera are: painful burning, with anxious sensations and compression in the region of the stomach, and in the region of the abdomen bordering upon it below; distension of the abdomen, with dreadful pains and disturbances in the bowels; frequent vomiting and diarrhœa, by which a yellowish, brownish, greenish fluid is evacuated with great violence. With these symptoms is combined a burning thirst for cold water and a rapid, but very small thread-like pulse.

These symptoms belong to the cholera, also when it is correctly treated with water.

In every medicinal, and in every false treatment, there arise as signs of a second and worse stadium, generally the following symptoms: Evacuations of a whey—or rice-water like fluid, with flakes which resemble cheese-mites; coldness of hands and feet, a changing of the color of the skin to a dirty pale yellow, to a bluish, and even to a blackish color; viciousness, flaccidness of the skin, and secretion of a tough, anxious perspiration; blackish color of the lips and nails; a death-like look, with deep sunken eyes, around which blackish rings form themselves; a hoarse inarticulate voice, a cold and light grey lead colored tongue; painful cramps in the limbs, especially in the calves of the legs and muscles of the belly; difficult groaning respiration, total cessation of urinary secretions, and of the vomiting and diarrhœa; a stupefied slumber, but without disturbance of the onsciousness; a tough, pitch-like disposition of the blood, a continual dwindling of the pulsations of the heart, increasing coldness of the skin—death.

(2) *The Nature of Disease in the Cholera* is a reaction of all the organs of digestion against matters of disease more in the cavities than in the walls of the organs, and an effort to cast off these matters through vomiting and purging.

An elucidation on this subject, of what nature these matters of disease may be, has not, as yet, been given in regard to the epidemic and Asiatic cholera; certain it is, however, that these matters are a consequence of a corruption of the elements, and thence also, of foods in general, and that they are the consequence especially of the corruption of the air. Whether the atmospheric corruption consists in its putrefaction or other chemical transformation, or whether in its impregnation with minute invisible animalculæ, thereupon I venture no opinion. The morbid matters which cause sporadic cholera, originate, partly, in a less extensive corruption of the elements; partly, and for the most part, in the consumption of corrupted foods. This corruption of the foods is of two kinds, either as having taken place before the foods were eaten, or, on the other hand, as originating in the digestive organs by reason of weakness, or chronic disease in those organs from poisons previously taken.

That to take either kind of cholera a predisposition is necessary, is evident for this reason, that even where the epidemic cholera is raging most violently, the great majority escape its attacks. The nature and causes of this predisposition are the same in general as those mentioned in the foregoing chapter.

The dysentery, as well as the cholera, may become a violent epidemic and apparently contagious; but they are, properly speaking, not contagious; in regard to contagiousness, these diseases may be denominated the transition diseases.

Whence is it, that sometimes the cholera does not set in with the initial symptoms of efforts at evacuation, but immediately with cramps and coldness of the extremities?

It comes from the relaxation and chronic illness of the digestive organs: it only occurs with such persons as have for a long time suffered in these organs. Through perverted diet, and especially from much doctoring, the stomach finally loses the power of free motion of the muscles, by which vomiting is produced. On the other hand, it is a proof of excellent health and strength of stomach, if it can immediately and without difficulty, rid itself, by vomiting, of an inimical substance, and immediately have a good appetite again—in like manner as a dog's stomach.

This same appearance manifests itself when cramps, without vomiting, sometimes ensue after medicinal vomitives are administered, and the reason is precisely the same. The stomach, too weak to eject the enemy, torments itself in endeavoring to do so, and this tormenting calls up the nervous convulsions of the cramp. In this manner a person may die of a vomitive, if vomiting does not ensue, a circumstance which has happened often enough.

This state of cramps and death-fear occurs in cholera as second stadium, also with those persons whose efforts at purification are disturbed and suppressed by medical interference. For the old method of cure, with its usual folly, combats the diarrhœa and vomiting, the very curative efforts of the disease: in this manner it has sacrificed far more victims than the malady itself.

(3) *The effect of the water-treatment* upon the cholera need not be specially shown, since it is similar to its effect on the dysentery. The burning thirst for cold water points out this drink in compliance with the infallibility of the human instinct, as the only and sovereign remedy. It cures by the dilution and reduction of the matters of disease, as also more especially by the elimination and ejection thereof through vomiting and evacuations.

If these two symptoms are still remaining, the water is applied as drink, as clyster, in sitz-baths, and wet compresses. If, however, these symptoms have already been suppressed through medical treatment, and if the second stadium, with the above-mentioned principal symptoms, is thus brought on, then the water must be directed, by means of the wet envelopments, strong rubbing of the feet, moderate drinking and bathing, towards exciting into action the energy of the skin, until this object be attained, whereupon, then, the water is applied again to the digestive organs.

(4) *The Effects of the Medical Treatment of Cholera.* —At first in the commencement of the disease oleaginous remedies are administered, of which I have already spoken. In the most direct contradiction to themselves the mediciners give now a remedy to stop the evacuation (and this is generally the case), now a remedy to excite vomiting. That the first manner of proceeding causes great injury is evident from former expositions. The second manner of proceeding is quite as injurious; for the medical vomitives consist of poisons which neither moderate nor dilute the matters of disease at hand, but have the contrary effect; they consist of poisons which do not dissolve the old mucous slime, but necessarily cause a fresh flow of mucus, because without this mucous protection the walls of the stomach and of the bowels would be corroded, and more or less destroyed through the operation of the poison.

In the cholera medicine has exhibited its injuriousness on a large scale; according to official accounts, of those attacked with the cholera in Russia, who, on account of their remoteness from physician and drug shop, were not medically, and, consequently, not at all, treated, not half so many died as of those treated medically. A like proportion to the discountenance of allopathy exhibits itself between homœopathic and allopathic treatment. It is also to be added and taken into consideration, that those cholera patients who survive the allopathic treatment, have always a long, oftentimes a life-long chronic malady to labor under, because the elimination of the cholera-humors is not promoted by medicine, but hindered and rendered quite impossible, and because to these humors the medicinal poisons are superadded and remain in the body more or less during life.

On the contrary, if a cholera-patient has not, as yet, taken any medicine, and if the alvine evacuations are still in operation, no chance of death is possible under correct water-treatment, and still less possible are after-pains and the origination of chronic illnesses.

XIV.

THE PRIMARY INFLAMMATORY DISEASES IN GENERAL.

REMARK.—By primary inflammation we understand that form of inflammation which the physicians call the acute, and also the synochous.

(1) *Symptoms of Primary Inflammation.*—In all inflammations of the internal parts, and in violent inflammations of the external parts, fever is present. In the inflamed part there is an universal increase of warmth even to heat, and an abnormal accumulation of blood, with which is necessarily combined a high red color. These accumulations of blood produce an enhanced fulness of the pulse, fill vessels with blood, which are otherwise bloodless, and cause a throbbing and palpitation in vessels where other-

wise no pulsation is to be perceived. In the inflamed part are pains frequently of a violent, shooting nature. Thus the primary or curative inflammation is distinguished from the secondary or destroying inflammation, by the heightened degree and rapid course of the former, but still in a greater degree and far more essentially, are the two kinds distinguished from each other *by the abnormally increased structural disposition of all primary inflammations;* while on the contrary, in the secondary inflammation this disposition never exceeds the normal energy, but often sinks below it, as this is especially the case in the typhus inflammation.

The only assistance which the hydriatic pathology can receive and make use of from the medical pathology, and indeed must make use of, is that part which treats of the symptoms of diseases; this must, however, be done with extreme caution and the full understanding of the subject, to prevent the transfer of many errors from the medical to the hydriatic pathology.

The above-enumerated symptoms of primary inflammation are to be found in the writings of the physicians, and they belong to this form of disease really and originally. But the symptoms of alteration in the disposition of the blood and the origination of false structures which the medical pathology ascribes also to the *inflammation*, belong solely to the *medical treatment* of this disease; they are an effect of medicine and the non-use of water, they are so foreign to the true form of inflammation in itself, that the slightest trace of such symptoms never appears, when the disease is treated from beginning to end with water.

(2) *The Nature of Disease in the Primary form of Inflammation* consists in a combat of the organism against

foreign acrid poisonous substances afloat in the system, set free from the mucous coatings of the stomach and bowels, or in heightened re-formative activity of the organism in cases of partial destructions of the organic structure from external violence, as in the case of wounds, burns, &c., &c.

The manner in which the body gets burdened with foreign and acrid matters through unwholesome diet or false method of cure, and how these matters enveloped in mucus lie for a length of time inactive and uninjurious, yet how they are released either by suppression of the insensible perspiration, by contraction of cold, or because the part of the body in which they lie renews itself, and thus loses the old, and endeavors to exude it—all this has been already set forth by me and demonstrated, and I can, therefore, enter upon the detail-account of the internal processes of inflammation.

The inflammation arising from external injuries remains here unconsidered, since they belong to the chapter upon surgical diseases.

Those substances which are at first introduced into the body as foreign and disease-causing, are commonly those proceeding from unwholesome diet, not medicinal substances.

The substances from false diet incapable of assimilation, arise in the excessive use of salt; the consumption of articles in the incipient stages of putrefaction, as for example, of strong cheese and rancid butter; in the use of sharp spices, as pepper; and in the use of alcoholic and intoxicating drinks. In consequence of the law, that the digestive organs can digest no substances which are sharper than the gastric juice and gall together, therefore, the above-mentioned sharp and acrid substances which are intermixed with the foods and drinks, pass unassimilated in their sharp acrid constitution, into the circulation, and through it into the whole body, while the other ingredients of the foods and drinks thus intermixed are digested and transformed into organic essence. When medicine is administered in a diarrhœa, or common indisposition, or in a contagious exanthematous disease, then actual poisons are introduced into the body in addition to the acrid sharp substances of the false diet. In such a manner a person may accumulate in himself a considerable quantity of sharp and poisonous matter, without ever having had an inflammatory disease, in the cure of which he has necessarily been medicinally poisoned.

As soon as these matters are, during a long and severe cold, released from their mucous fetters, they produce violent pains, by coming in contact with the nerves. If the organism is not vigorous enough to undertake the effort of radically eliminating the matters, these pains continue for a long time, return frequently, and are called rheumatic pains. If, however, the organism has the strength necessary to undertake its radical cure, it carries on still more extensively the work of releasing the peccant matter by dissolving the old mucus, and does not again envelop the released foreign matters in fresh mucus, but forces great quantities of blood into that organ, in which they are in greatest quantity present. Abnormal quantities of blood are there necessary for several purposes, to wit, first, to dissolve more and more the old phlegmy mucus, to drive the released poisonous matters towards the skin, to protect the nerves and other organic structures as much as possible against the destructive power of the poisons, which are carried past them towards the skin; and second, *to restore by new formations* the partial destructions which still are necessarily produced in organic structures, for which purpose much blood is requisite; for blood is the material from which the vital energy creates all organic structures.

From this necessity of re-formation of organic destructions, the abnormally strong re-formative disposition of the primary inflammatory disease explains itself in the simplest and clearest manner, which indeed has hitherto been a riddle to all pathologists.

The blood is the material which forms all organic structures, but these formations cannot proceed in a normal and organically perfect manner without oxygen sufficient to the transformation of the fluid blood into solid organic parts, and they cannot proceed without hydrogen to change the refuse solid parts into transpirable fluid. These two materials are the constituent parts of water. In the inflammatory form of disease the body needs for the above-mentioned purposes these two materials in an abnormal quantity. *Without sufficient support from these two materials, the abnormally heightened re-formative disposition of the system cannot elaborate to organic perfectness the organic new formations of destroyed parts, but it must necessarily produce mal-formations—and those are the false formations of the inflammatory form of disease,* which physicians cannot explain to themselves, and which always arise when the skin and stomach are not supplied with as much water as the instinct requires—unless directly in its commencement the inflammation is suppressed by repeated blood-lettings, of which I shall speak more fully and particularly.

The fever, which attends every violent inflammation, finds its explanation in the abnormally, and far above the normal energies, elevated activity of the organism, and in the abnormally increased consumption of oxygen.

(3) *The effects of the hydriatic treatment on the primary form of Inflammation,* have been given already under section 2, in all the points of chief moment. For the complete dissolution of all foreign matters in the inflamed part the blood requires copious dilution, so that it may penetrate into the minutest spaces, and possess the greatest possible dissolvent power; to expedite the foreign matters towards the skin it requires an uncommon quantity of transpirable matter, to which the water furnishes partly the material, and partly the means; finally, the pores of the skin, in order to eliminate the offending matters, require frequent and repeated cleansing, and the refreshing, cooling, strengthening influence which water exercises upon that organ.

So much upon the requisiteness of water for the purpose of excreting foreign matters; the indispensableness of water for the purpose of rebuilding organical destruction, has already been considered under division 2.

(4) *The effects of the medical treatment upon Inflammatory Disease,* are diametrically contrary to the effects of the hydriatic.

Under the water-treatment the instinct is appeased and satisfied, under the medical treatment it is maltreated; for, in every primary inflammation the patient has most parching thirst for water, both in the skin and the tongue, and has in every disease, and in every condition, the greatest disgust for medicine and poison; under the water-cure the symptoms of disease are moderated, but still sustained, until the purpose of the inflammation has been gained; under the medical treatment the symptoms, as efforts of the organism to cure itself, are suppressed, and the re-construction of organic demolitions is rendered impossible. Under the medical treatment an actual cure is a physiological impossibility; still, through medicinal means and appliances, a deliverance from death, with some exceptions, is most generally possible in this disease. Bleeding especially is their most efficacious remedy. Thus, if, in that stadium of the disease wherein the blood has not as yet passed into corruption, recourse is had to sufficient bleedings, the quantity of blood necessary to an inflammation is thus withdrawn from the inflamed organ, and the inflammation must for this reason cease. Often enough the patient then dies of debilitation from loss of blood, but it is more frequently the case, that he does not die, while, on the contrary, he almost always dies, if neither water nor medical assistance (under this head I include blood-lettings) is administered.

Such, however, is the dreadful effect of blood-letting and poisons upon the inflammatory form of disease, that where death does not ensue, they always leave a chronic malady, which is, in most cases, far worse than death itself. As a rule, we find it mentioned in all medical therapies, that the medically cured inflammations generally leave a weakness in the inflamed part, which continues through the remainder of life. This is not by far the most disastrous effect of the medical treatment; it happens very frequently that it is followed sometimes sooner, sometimes later, by chronic ulcerations, indurations which grow to cartilage, false growths, schirrous exanthem, which finally turns to cancer, the accumulation of an abnormal quantity of serous liquid, and even mortification. These after-effects of medically treated inflammation, we find mentioned in all medical instruction books. The manner in which such destructive diseases arise, finds a general explanation in my expositions already given ; further on, when the secondary diseases are treated of, I will give the detail demonstrations.

The poisons are less effectual in suppressing inflammatory symptoms than the abstractions of blood. Still, the former afford the latter great assistance. More recently mercury, in its various preparations, is almost always employed as an antiphlogistic medicament, besides a mass of other poisons.

When poison is introduced into the stomach, that organ must either cast it out immediately, or envelope it in mucus. To accomplish the first of these purposes requires much more energy than the second. Sometimes the medicament heightens the symptoms, and produces new, although other symptoms ; sometimes it quiets them ; the first is the case when the organism attempts to throw off the poison of the medicine, the last when it envelopes it, and tolerates it within itself. On suitable repetition of the doses of poison the organism is always driven to the latter expedient.

That the symptoms of disease, if they be curative, and consequently voluntary symptoms, must abate, when an uncommon exercise of power is demanded in another organ, is of itself evident ; the power of inflammation in another organ must abate exactly in accordance with the proportion of strength employed to generate mucus in the digestive organs. Hence, it is evident, that the poisons depress or entirely suppress the inflammatory symptoms.

The effect of medical treatment upon primary inflammations is accordingly either death from debilitation, or the origination of chronic complaints; for this reason, that in the first place neither the original peccant matter of the disease is eliminated by the medical treatment, nor can the organic destructions be restored through new formations; that, secondly, new poisons are brought into the body, and firmly fixed there in mucous envelopment; and that, thirdly, the general organism is debilitated by the abstraction of blood, and most especially the nerves are affected. A nervous disorder is often enough brought on by repeated copious bleedings, and then insanity follows in the train of consequences.

Sometimes the mere quenching of the thirst with water suffices to cure an inflammatory disease; however death frequently follows such a simple treatment, and it very rarely cures the malady radically. But the appliances of the methodic hydriatique cures radically under all circumstances every primary inflammation with uncommon despatch, and a chance of death is absolutely impossible, if the water be employed in the very commencement of it.

The primary form of inflammation is the purest and most energetic curative form of the human organism, it has been growing more and more seldom for a number of years, and the nervous form of disease more and more frequent. That is the effect of a method of cure, which borrows all its remedies from the armories of death, the torture and the executioner's agents—poison, fire, steel—these three words comprehend the whole "apparatus medicaminum" of the art of mischief, as reason calls it, which is a devouring cancer on the marrow of the human race, and which, by newly invented arts of a medical Jesuitism, gives itself all imaginable trouble to induce the magistracy or rulers of the country to suppress the true system of cure.

XV.

INFLAMMATION OF THE EYES—INFLAMMATION OF THE BRAIN—INFLAMMATION OF THE THROAT, OR QUINSY—INFLAMMATION OF THE LUNGS.

(1) *Inflammation of the Eyes* falls into many subdivisions, according to the degree of violence (taraxis, chemosis, ophthalmia), and the different parts of the eye, which are particularly the seat of the inflammation (inflammation of the sockets of the eye, of the eyelids, of the eyeballs, of the cornea, of the iris, &c., &c). All these, and a number of other subdivisions, are in the hydriatic practice not only superfluous, but unnecessarily perplexing, and productive of confusion, and may be entirely disregarded. Therefore we will use here only the general term of Inflammation of the Eyes.

When the organism endeavors by acute efforts to throw off foreign, acrid, poisonous matter from the eyes by means of secretions of mucus from the glands and glandules, it can effect this only by an abnormally heightened energy of action, which is here almost entirely local, and consequently not without abnormal accumulation of blood and increase of warmth. If the heat be not cooled, and the eyes not bathed with water, the quality of the blood becomes altered, and false formations arise, which are of various kinds; oftentimes a film grows over the eye-ball, and produces blindness.

Inflammations of the eyes particularly are sometimes epidemic, for instance in Egypt, when the wind, impregnated with fine sand, drives it into the eyes, and in large towns, when a dry heat prevails in the summer season; and consequently the fine stone-dust, which the wheels of a thousand vehicles grind from the stone pavement, is not kept down by rain or moisture, as, for instance, in Berlin. Allopathy administers its antiphlogistica, applies leeches and Spanish flies, and smears poisonous salves, wherein mercury again plays a principal part, into that delicate noble organ of the sight. Whoever has, in such a manner, passed through the executioners' hands, has before him a threefold prospect; first, always and unconditionally chronic decrease of the keenness of vision, which usually soon grows to such weakness as to incapacitate the eyes for any in-door business; second, in most cases a permanent life-long redness, periodical prickling or pains in the eyes, and nightly suppuration; third, in very many instances after the expiration of a number of years, blindness from decay of the visual nerve.

It is evident, from the former deductions of this book, how the poison rubbed into and through coercive means imbibed by the eyes may for a series of years be held in confinement, and it can at last still destroy the visual nerve. Blindness may come on twenty years and more after such a treatment, and yet the cause in material substance is still that same poison which so long afterwards destroys the nerve of sight.

In Berlin, as a chief seat of inflammation of eyes and of allopathy, many hundreds have in this way been deprived of their sight by the most celebrated physicians, and even now not a single year passes in which such victims are not sacrificed to the night of blindness.

If water be rightly applied in eye-baths and wet bandages directly in the commencement of the acute stadium, the purification of the eyes will be soon effected, and no after-affections can in anywise possibly ensue. If, after the eyes have been injured by poisonous applications, in addition to the above-named appliance, the douche, back-head bath, and foot-bath be employed, the acute crisis will again return, and by perseverance the former keenness of sight, provided that the organism is still possessed of good age and vital energy.

(2) *Inflammation of the Brain* comprises the inflammation both of the brain and of the membrane covering the brain, and a distinction between them is entirely unnecessary in the hydriatic system.

The symptoms of this disease are glaring red eyes, a fixed, staring, or wild rolling look; the blood-vessels of the head are greatly dilated, and beat violently under the influence of a high general fever; the skin is dry. A stupefying, oppressive feeling in the head is followed by a fixed violent pain, which is increased by every strong impression of the mind, and which at times runs into torpid, at times into raging deliria.

We have here excluded external injuries as an originating cause.

The nature of this disease consists in a violent reaction of the organism against foreign matter in the brain, which is set free from its mucous envelopment by colds in the head, by a systematic water-cure in chronic affections of the brain, by abnormal determination of blood to the parts, brought on by excessive exertion and application of the mind.

The effects of the hydriatic treatment upon inflammations of the brain are elimination of the matter of disease, partly through perspiration and eruptions on the head, but more through abnormal secretions from the alvearies or hollows of the ears, and from the nostrils (catarrh); oftentimes these secretions have quite an abnormal color and acridness.

Under the water-treatment, inflammation of the brain cannot possibly event either in death or in the foundation of any secondary affection of the head.

The effects of the medical treatment upon inflammation of the brain, are either death under apoplectic and convulsive circumstances, and palsy of the brain, or a sensible enfeeblement of that organ, or secondary brain-disease, as chronic inflammation, gradual ulceration of the brain, accumulation of serous liquid, softening of the brain, finally also insanity.

(3) *Inflammation of the Throat, or Sore Throat.*—By sore throat we intend sometimes all inflammations of the various organs and parts of the throat, at other times only the inflammations of the wind-pipe, and again also the inflammations of the contiguous parts.

Besides the fore-mentioned general symptoms of inflammation, that of the wind-pipe is attended by a cough, of a hoarse and barking tone, that of the œsophagus with difficulties in swallowing.

When death does not ensue under the medical treatment, still after-affections always do, which, in favorable cases, consist in a predisposition to fresh attacks of inflammation of the throat; in unfavorable cases, however, in a chronic inflammation of the organs that were affected, further in indurations and ossifications of the wind-pipe and œsophagus, further in origination of schirrus and cancer.

(4) *The Inflammation of the Lungs, and Diaphragm,* have like symptoms, and are treated alike in the water-cure.

Violent compression of the breast, and difficulties in breathing, with high fever, a pain in the breast, which now is dull, now piercing, hot breath and expectoration of phlegm, and frequently, also, of blood, are the symptoms of inflammation of the lungs.

The results of the hydriatic as well as of the medical treatment correspond to the same results in the other inflammations. In the water-treatment actual cure is effected through the critical discharges of the cough, and in general also of boils; in the medical treatment the aforementioned after-evils arise, and, in particular, in the last instance of inflammation of the lungs and chest, ulceration of the lungs, commonly called consumption, sets in.

The inflammation of the other parts of the body, as of the liver, of the tongue, of the diaphragm, of the stomach, of the matrix, &c., are analogous to those just described, as well in regard to the symptoms, and condition, and nature of the disease, as in regard to the effects which the water-cure and medicine exert upon them respectively; still each is variously modified according to the different construction and function of the different organs. The very limited space which I can still allow to primary inflammations I must devote to the consideration of the metastases.

When, as is generally the case, matters of disease are present in several organs of one and the same body, and are set free from their envelopment of mucus by a severe cold or other cause, still, then, a genuine and energetic inflammation cannot take place but in a single organ, because the organism in general does not possess vigor sufficient to a victorious encounter of the inflammatory struggle in two different organs; exceptions occur very rarely, and only in uncommonly strong organisms, well observed, I speak only of primary, violent, and genuine inflammations, not of rheumatic, still less of chronic inflammations. It is no contradiction of this position, that the adjoining parts and organs are also somewhat affected by the inflammations; for these affections arise only from a lateral influence of the spontaneously inflamed organ, and must follow from the consensuality of contiguous organs.

Another circumstance not to be confounded with the position just considered, is the transplantation of the inflammation from one organ to another, and always to a nobler organ, and one more influential, and possessing more power over life. These transplantations of a disease, and especially of an inflammatory, is called a metastasis (genuine metastasis).

Metastasis is generally the effect of a false medical treatment. Genuine metastasis is produced only by freshly contracted cold; false metastasis arises from medicinal poisoning.

A true metastasis I call such as is produced by a violently altered direction of the humors, and especially of the transpiratory faculty; the violence which this produces consists seldom in colds taken in the usual manner, but so much the more frequently in a false application of cold water, and still more of ice. If the cooling water compresses, or local baths of cold water, are continued too long, without in the meantime allowing the organism the space and means for reaction by the application of warming cold-water-bandages, the fluid of the insensible perspiration is forced into other organs, and there sets free matters of disease, and thus causes fresh inflammation. The original inflammation in the former organ must abate, because the organism has not powers sufficient to two simultaneous inflammations; consequently, the organism must again envelope in mucus the peccant matter set free in the first inflamed organ. In such a manner, by the false application of water, an inflammation of the bowels may be transmitted to the chest, as also inflammation of the chest to the brain. When physicians, according to their method, make water-applications in inflammations, they take it always too cold, and continue its influence too long, so that they almost always produce metastasis; they make use, also, of ice, which must be wholly excluded from the true water-cure system. Under correct water-treatment, a metastasis is impossible, and the directions for such water-treatment can be given so simply and clearly, that even the most uninformed cannot err, when he has read them.

The false metastasis I call that transposition of the inflammation which is produced by poisonous substances in another organ recently introduced into the body. When, for instance, mustard plasters are applied behind the ears or upon the back for inflamed eyes, then this is a false metastasis, which is intentionally produced by the physicians, as a so-called derivative. Frequently they accomplish the same end unintentionally, but quite in the same manner, by poisons administered internally. It is clear that the primary inflammation of an organ must somewhat abate when inflammation and impostumation is produced elsewhere by corrosive drugs, and the powers of the body are thereby divided ; and it is just as clear that the peccant matter of the primarily inflamed organ is not thereby eliminated, but that fresh poisonous matters are introduced into the artificially inflamed organ.

The real metastasis is distinguished by its greater energy and marked primary character from the false metastasis, which, in most cases, partakes somewhat of the character of the chronic and lingering inflammation, and sometimes passes over into such.

XVI.

COUGHS AND COLDS.

These are diseases of the most general and simple kind, and, in the commencement, are always curative endeavors to eliminate peccant matter by means of secretions of mucus. In persons afflicted with chronic diseases they lose their primary and curative character, and degenerate into various secondary forms, as for instance, into obstructed catarrh, into the dry cough, which, with some, produces chronic affection of the throat, and is the forerunner of ulceration of the lungs. Here, we have only to do with the primary forms, which are not of long duration, and cause copious secretion of mucus.

The excretions of the brain, that is, the refuse substance of the brain, as well as also foreign and poisonous matters, which have found their way into the brain through the circulation of the blood, are discharged mostly through the nostrils in the mucus and phlegm of the nose, less from the ears, in the form of earwax, least of all, and indeed only in sickness, from the sockets of the eyes. Primary catarrh is thus a secretion of acrid foreign humor from the brain, and the inflammation of the mucous membrane of the nose is produced by the acrid and corrosive power of the foreign humors coming in contact with it. Allopathy, which, in its usual superficial manner, confounds the symptoms and even the effects of the disease, with the nature of the disease, endeavors to find the *nature* of catarrh in an inflammation of the mucous membrane of the nose, while the inflammation is only an *effect* of the catarrh, and its nature consists in a cleansing of the brain. Colds are usually the occasion of the origination of this cleansing, inasmuch as they release the foreign matters encased in mucus, whereupon, then, the purifying effort commences. The feeling, alone, tells every one that the cause and seat of the cold does not lie in the mucous glands of the nose only, but still more in the brain also, since in the beginning of the cold, confusedness in the head, and after it has passed off, a pleasurable sensation and increased ease of the brain is experienced, which manifests itself also in the ease and perspicuity of thought which in the commencement of the cold is very much restricted.

All the circumstances and processes, together with the causes of primary cough, are quite analogous with those of catarrh. In a like superficial manner, allopathy declares its nature to be an inflammation of the mucous glands of the throat, while its nature consists really in the elimination of foreign matters from the lungs.

It is a real pleasure to see how primary coughs and

colds, under the water-treatment, increase their secretions of phlegm, mucus, and expectoration, and are thus cured so much the more quickly.

In the water-cure, obstructed catarrh becomes loose and flowing, and in the same manner precisely, dry cough, pains and strictures of the breast, are changed to critical cough, by which the phlegm-enveloped matters are thrown off, since otherwise, at a later period of life, they would have caused ulceration or dropsy on the chest.

The acridness of the secretions in catarrhs and coughs, which, in the case of the former, is oftentimes so corroding that they painfully affect the nostrils, and even the contiguous part of the upper lip, and give them a high inflamed red color, proves sufficiently, that the secreted phlegm contains matters which are quite distinct from the phlegm itself, which, as is well known, is a perfectly mild substance, free from all taste and smell.

In the wide field of disease the group of the inflammatory forms of disease borders upon the group of the rheumatic forms, and, in individual cases of disease, one may be in doubt under which of these groups they are to be classed. Also, primary coughs and catarrhs are oftentimes intermediate forms between those two groups.

XVII.

INTERMITTING FEVER.

Fevers are usually classified under three main heads—capillary fever, intermitting fever, and nervous fever. The capillary fevers are subdivided into primary and secondary; to the former belong the inflammatory fevers;

to the latter belong the typhus and putrid. The catarrhal and rheumatic fevers form a transition or intermediate class, and, according as they partake more of the inflammatory or more of the nervous character, incline at one time to the primary capillary form, at another time to the nervous form.

Of all fevers only the primary capillary fevers and the intermitting fever belong always to the primary diseases; generally, the catarrhal fevers belong there also, to whose more minute consideration room fails us in this edition; they are among the most unimportant and best known diseases, and their nature is apparent from the chapters on the inflammatory and rheumatic forms of disease.

The symptoms of a corrupt or diseased stomach in a fever give it that character which is usually called gastric. In the pure inflammatory form of disease all gastric character is wanting; on the contrary, the gastric character accompanies the intermitting fever, and is the over-ruling and most prominent. The intermitting fever is distinguished from the gastric catarrhal fever by the regular cessation of the former for a space of time, after which it returns again; there is an intermitting fever, which returns every day, one which returns every second day, and one which returns every third day. There are also intermitting fevers, which for certain periods of time set in twice a day.

(1) *Symptoms of the Intermitting Fever.*—The preceding oftentimes very severe chill, which in the inflammatory as well as intermitting fever, I do not include among the symptoms of recognition or distinction, because it is no characteristicum, and moreover, because I do not con-

sider it as belonging to the disease itself, but only as a preparation for it.

The symptoms of intermitting fever are: blue color of the lips and nails, scanty secretion of water-colored urine, and a small rapid pulse during the period of the chill. During the heat, which generally extends itself downwards, the pulse beats full and quick, but still hard; the urine takes a clear light-red coloring; the head is disturbed, and a feeling of faintness arises from the stomach. The dry heat is followed by perspiration, and the pulse becomes softer; the perspiration has always an unpleasant, commonly a sour smell, and the urine precipitates a considerable sediment if it is kept standing for some time in a glass vessel. During all the described stadia the patient has a strong thirst for cold water, and in the course of the perspiration period feels, also, a strong desire for a water-bath.

(2) *The Nature of Intermitting Fever* consists in impurity of the stomach, in the energy of the skin being partially destroyed by the presence of matters of disease under it, *and in a reaction of the organism against these morbific matters.* The fever is an effort to throw off, by perspiration from the skin, the morbific matters under it; the great thirst during the periods of the chill, which does not appear in the chill preceding inflammatory diseases, does not arise from the want of an abnormal quantity of oxygen for new formations, but merely from the want of a dissolving fluid, and is a proof of the effort of the organism to dissolve slimy corrupted substances in the stomach, and then, with the assistance of water, to discharge them by vomiting or diarrhœa.

The cause of intermitting fevers lies in the corruption

of the stomach, which is produced sometimes by unwholesome diet, sometimes by the contamination of the atmosphere and water by the presence of malaria in the neighborhood of swamps and low lands, and sometimes by the conjoint effect of both these pernicious causes.

(3) *The Effects of Water-treatment* on the intermitting fever is actual cure of the disease through diarrhœa, vomiting, and secretion of critical perspiration, and critical urine. The water taken through the stomach into the circulation sets free from mucous envelopment the matters of disease deposited in the flesh, and conducts them to the skin in the fluid, which passes off in insensible perspiration. The bath invigorates the skin, cleanses it, keeps the pores open, and, by means of the reaction after the bath, conducts the current of the juices from the internal parts towards the skin.

Although the water-cure, when it is applied in good season, as first treatment, always cures the intermitting fever radically, yet it is not effected so rapidly as with the inflammatory fevers, because the intermitting fever is a compound disease, and because there is no curative form of disease so pure and energetic as the inflammatory form.

(4) *The Effect of Medical Treatment.*—Here, as ever, the medical treatment suppresses the symptoms of disease, and thereby converts the primary disease into a secondary, i. e. ends in the chronic fixture of the matters of disease. The fever remedies of the mediciners are China, Belladonna, Arsenic. Since the curative efforts in this fever originate chiefly in the stomach, it must naturally desist from these efforts, when substances, that are very injurious to it, are thrown into it and paralyse its energies.

Then the curative symptoms of the fever naturally cease, and the mediciners, when they have suppressed the curative symptoms of a primary disease, think or say, they have cured the disease. The patient's own feelings enlighten them always to the contrary; the feeling and instinct of the patient never err in primary diseases, and never deceive; physiology and true pathology speak likewise to the contrary, and the later after-effects of such medicinal cures teach in a terrible manner the contrary.

The medical remedies always dispel the intermitting fever for a time; however, it frequently returns again, as soon as the organism has somewhat recovered from the poisoning. Then medicine is administered anew, which often enough converts the curative fever into a destroying disease, into mucous fever, even into a putrid fever. These changes produced by medical treatment take place without any perceptible interval of health. After such intervals, and sometimes not till a number of years afterwards, in consequence of the medical treatment there set in ossification of the stomach, dropsy, enlargements of the liver, besides contraction of the heart, and many other of such like destroying diseases.

In intermitting fever the diet must be modified according to certain rules; in all those primary diseases treated of before the intermitting fever, the instinct is the only and infallible regulator of the diet. The intermitting fever forms in this, as in many other respects, a transition from the primary to the secondary diseases.

XVIII.

CONCLUDING REMARKS ON PRIMARY DISEASES.

ALTHOUGH the directions for all the practical forms of application of water against diseases, together with the rules for the diet, belong in a therapy, and consequently must be excluded from this work, still the statement of the practical *fundamental* rules is in its proper place in a pathology, because the establishment of the therapeutic foundation must be thence derived.

The colder the water, the stronger is the reaction of that part of the body which is brought in contact with it; the colder it is, so much the more does it accelerate the circulation of the blood, and thereby arouse all the energies of the excited organ to an abnormal height. Because now in all fevers there is already an abnormal excitation of the circulation, therefore the application of cold water in the form of full bath or entire ablution is injurious, and water of a temperature of from 57° to, at the highest, 77° Fah., must be used. *At least one should be aware, that the fever is increased by cold water, by tepid water however it is reduced;* the reduction is caused through the chemical effect of the water, the excitation through the dynamic effect of the cold. Exceptions may occur, wherein the experienced water-physician finds it expedient to elevate still higher the degree of fever, and accordingly applies cold water for a time, but an inexperienced person should never venture on this, and, in general, to avoid many accidents, it is necessary that the above be considered fundamental rules.

With such absolute infallibility does the instinct in all

primary diseases indicate the proper mode of application, that in fevers it manifests a disrelish to quite cold water, even where the patient has been accustomed to it previous to the fever, and his instinct was then fond of it.

When I now conclude the treatise on primary diseases, I do not mean to infer that I have in anywise exhausted the subject, but refer you to the title-page, which promises only the outlines of a pathology.

N.

THE SECONDARY OR DESTROYING DISEASES.

I.

GENERAL PRELIMINARY OBSERVATIONS.

ALTHOUGH the revision which I have undertaken with the division on primary diseases, has attained, neither in extent of material, nor in its order and arrangement, that degree of perfection which I should have achieved with more leisure for authorship; still, I am compelled by many circumstances, in the revision of the division treating of secondary diseases, to hold myself still more to the surface, and to publish again this section with less alterations in its original form, and in its original contents.

As there are everywhere individuals and groups of transition between the classes of things created by human ingenuity, so is this also the case with every conceivable classification of disease. If more at leisure, I would have devoted a particular section to the transition group; now I must content myself with specifying as such the varieties of disease which compose this group, without setting apart a place for them in this work.

II.

THE MANNER IN WHICH THE THREE STADIA OF SECONDARY DISEASES ARISE.

In the division on primary diseases, it has already been shown, how poisonous and medicinal substances convert the primary diseases into secondary diseases.

False diet is generally cöoperative in the development of secondary disease. By this I mean the use of sharp, high-seasoned foods, and alcoholic drinks; furthermore, the want of bodily exercise, living in unwholesome and corrupted atmosphere, as is too frequently found in the habitations of the poor, and the consumption of proportionately too much food. Whoever has not a healthy stomach, should never fully satisfy his appetite; furthermore, he also should not, who leads a sedentary life, even if he has a strong stomach—one departure from nature's laws necessitates *another*. It is contrary to nature not to satisfy the appetite; it is contrary to nature to lead a sedentary life.

Only such an one as has a strong stomach, and at the same time takes much bodily exercise, may be allowed to *fully satiate his appetite*, provided he pursues a water-diet.

Other cöoperating causes, which aid in laying the foundation of secondary diseases, are the over-exertion of individual organs, especially of the brain and the generative organ, and also mental affections of a violent and melancholy nature.

A disturbance in the balance of the circulation and in other functions is produced by the long continued false and partial use of cold water. Whoever, for instance, washes head and face daily in cold water, and the feet never, or but very seldom, must sooner or later suffer of cold feet, and generally, also, of repletion of blood, and excess of heat in the head. In common life we are accustomed to call this, which arises from the false circulation of the blood, "plethora, or excess of blood;" but the opinion which gives rise to this is an entirely false one. A disease of plethora, i. e. a disease arising from *too much blood,* does not exist, but this apparent disease consists always in *false* and *unequal* circulation of the blood. The only remedy for this complaint lies in cold water; but for this purpose it must be applied precisely in the contrary manner to that which the doctors suppose and recommend.

Secondary disease has three several stadia, which, indeed, in the reality are not nicely demarcated, but flow into each other by a gradual transition.

The first stadium is the period of oft-returning efforts of the body to produce anew an acute disease wherewith to cure itself; these efforts, however, never succeed in full without aid from the water-cure. In this stadium acute pains frequently arise, which end either in a hot and red tumor, for instance, with toothache and other rheumatic affections, or find vent in abnormal secretions of mucus and phlegm from the nose, windpipe, eyes, throat, bowels; or, with those who are more successful, in driving out boils and eruptions. All these various forms are decided signs that the body is still possessed of inclination and strength to cure itself; but it has no more the power to accomplish this cure through a general and radical reaction, through a properly acute disease, but attempts to gain it little by little, by means of acute-like partial efforts frequently repeated. If a fresh attack lays hold of the organism, generally from contraction of cold, still, then, it always reacts against it with acute pains.

When the painful curative struggles of the first stadium are suppressed by medicine, then the organism enters into

The second chronic stadium of disease, which is an apparent condition of tolerable health and is a state of quiet. In this period the organism has no longer strength enough to attempt its cure of its own accord, still enough, however, to hold the enveloped fettered morbific matters in statu quo. If, in this stadium, inimical influences act upon the body, it does not endeavor any more to react and eject the enemy, but simply endeavors to envelope it and fix it temporarily in mucus, that it may work no immediate effect on the animal economy. For this reason the former acute pains, which, indeed, are nothing else than the battle-music of the curative strife, die away, and, in lieu thereof, succeed disagreeable, dull, oppressed, nervous conditions, in which the patient feels a longing desire after acute pains. Instead of the symptoms of pain, which have now passed off, two others, much worse, have taken their place; first, diminished strength and energy of the whole machine, and second, the consciousness of the patient, that tells him, things are not as they should be in his body, an enemy is lurking there, the germ of death is forming, and bestirring itself apace.

In the second stadium there comes on not seldom a corpulence of a very notorious kind, that embonpoint of superfœtation with its peculiarly tumid and impotent expression, accompanied, generally, with baldness and decay of the fire of the eye. If then a little French rouge is added to the cheeks, the tout ensemble appears like a caricature on a healthy man; like a plump, well-stuffed doll.

Still, the patient, in the second chronic stadium, can attend to his business tolerably well, and he passes generally for healthy, because he is large and fat, and has no acute symptoms.

The third stadium is that of annihilation, either of the individual organs and senses, when the disease is only local, or of life itself, when it is general; or, indeed, of those organs which condition life. In the latter case the stadium is a slow, horrid, chronic dying, whose struggles and pains may be prolonged several years.

In this third period the organism is no longer possessed of powers and juices enough continually to curb, by mucous envelopment, the indwelling inimical humors; therefore, getting released, they begin internally to corrode, and ulcerate first in those organs and parts of the body where they are the most accumulated. Thus, then, originate the chronic ulcerations of individual internal organs, of the lungs, of the liver, of the stomach, &c. In this manner caries originate, and the so-called fistulas and cancers; in like manner arises the dissolution of the walls of the blood-vessels, which, in case of the larger arteries, causes death. Thus arises also the organic deformations and organic defects (of course the innate deformities excepted), cartilaginous growths, ossifications, polypi, and growths of all kinds solely through the effects of poison.

Many diseases of the third period may set in directly after a poisoning, without the foregoing first two stadia, if the poisoning has been carried by bunglers beyond the rules of the medical art.

In the third stadium belongs the chronic, pale, and cold swelling called dropsy. (See farther on the process of origination of this disease.)

It is, indeed, possible that a chronic complaint may arise through one or more of the afore-mentioned faults of diet; but it is an *extremely seldom case* in which this occurs without the co-operation of a medicinal poisoning.

Whoever, in an acute disease, has taken an *energetic*, powerful medicine, has been deprived of the possibility of dying a natural death from old age; he must, sooner or later, die a painful death from a secondary disease; unless, through water-cure and water-diet, he heals himself of the poisoning, and bears a new body.

You who read this book, if ever the deep-colored cup of poison is tendered you, cast it from you, mindful of this warning—that what you drink to-day will, in after years, bring upon you a miserable death by disease.

Are my deductions upon the after-deadly effects of poison not evident enough to carry conviction to the mind of every one? Do they still require the corroboration of instances and cases? Alas! of them there is no lack.

The secret medicinal consultee Toffana, in Naples, knew how to graduate her doses so as to cause the death of the victims to her skill in any required space of time, just according to the desire of her applicants, either immediately, or in one year, or in ten years. This woman was a medical genius, and certainly she would have "cured" any acute disease, according to the rules of art, with her nice remedies, because it was an easy matter for her to mete out the requisite dose. Also, many of the victims of Brinvilliers and Gesche Timm died of one of the above-mentioned secondary diseases many years after having been poisoned.

I should be sorry if, despite all that has been said, some one should reply to me, "these secret murderesses gave poison, the physicians, however, give medicine."

Abstractedly from the point, that poison is identical with medicine, according to every definition affecting their nature and their essence (the only difference that exists does not lie in the thing itself, but in the intention; if one gives poison to cause mischief, then it is called poison; if one gives it under the erroneous opinion of curing with it, then it is called medicine), and also that the intention of the agent makes no alteration in the nature of the matter, then the physicians, in all energetic acute diseases, administer poisons, even according to the most restricted nomenclature, by which only the destroying poisons receive the name of poisons: they give arsenic, mercury, belladonna, prussic acid; in short, they exhaust the whole arsenal of death.

III.

THE CURE OF THE SECONDARY DISEASES.

As the causes of the perfect diseases are foreign matters in the suffering organism, which must be eliminated, therefore, a true cure can only be effected through the activity of the organism, aided by the dissolvent power of water, whereby skin and stomach are raised to the condition of greatest reaction and activity.

In acute diseases physic blinds the eye of a short-sighted observer with the appearance of cure, which the poisoning, by suppression of symptoms, spreads over its mischievous work; but in chronic diseases it no longer commands the ability to dazzle, and it confesses its weakness.

The water-cure cures all secondary diseases of the first and second stadium with the most perfect certainty. (Concerning the method of cure of Priessnitz, and the internal process of healing in chronic complaints, see the work entitled, "Spirit of the Graefenberg Water-Cure, by J. H. Rausse.")

Whoever, in the first stadium, enters a water-cure establishment, may expect a cure as speedy as radical, because his body still, of its own accord, presses on to the crisis and cure.

Whoever, in the second stadium, enters upon the water-cure, must determine upon a long course of treatment, because he requires a considerable length of time, to be restored to the condition of the first stadium, whereupon, then, the cure is certain. By perseverance he will be radically cured of all his afflictions and diseased humors, and regains not only his former healthfulness, but also his strength of body.

Patients, in the third stadium, are only partially and conditionally curable, and they must always undergo such a long and irksome course of treatment, that they may well consider, beforehand, their capability and determination of perseverance.

The first condition of curableness is, that sufficient vital energy be still left; and the second, that ulceration of the lungs has not yet commenced. Subject, then, to these two provisions the hydriatic system cures, of the far-advanced ulcerations of internal organs, only those of the mouth, of the œsophagus, of the stomach, and of the bowels, because here the water can be directly applied to the diseased part through drinking and clysters. Of cancerous ulcers, those which are external and in the stomach and bowels are curable ; fistulas are cured ; farthermore, all external chronic suppurations, which are a sign of good constitution, because the organism has strength to drive the poisoned humors to the external surface. Farther, caries are curable, and also the dissolution of the walls of the blood-vessels in its commencement, the diseased affections of all the senses, if their nerves are not yet entirely destroyed. Deaf and blind persons have, in Graefenberg, regained an acute hearing and keen sight. Finally, dropsy is curable in its commencement.

All these patients must determine to persist in a course of treatment for one year and upwards. The cure requires so much more time, the deeper the roots of the disease have penetrated, and extended throughout the organism ; and especially according to the number of complaints combined in one body.

It is not advisable to force the cure with such patients, and endeavor to extort an early crisis. Before this is possible, a considerable time must be spent in invigorating and regaining vital energy, except where the organism is still unimpaired, and the complaint only local. Generally, it is not expedient to sweat such a patient every day until the crisis comes ; rather it will be most advisable to alternate frequently the water-diet with the proper water-cure in suitable periods.

Many such patients have left Graefenberg without being radically cured, satisfied with the progress they had made, and the great alleviation and invigoration they had obtained, forced away from the water-cure establishment through impatience and lack of perseverance, or on account of uncontrollable circumstances.

IV.

LOSS OF APPETITE. HEARTBURN AND ERUCTATIONS. HARD AND SLUGGISH STOOL. THE FALSE OR UNREAL MUCUS. WORMS.

Constant loss of Appetite may have its cause in two different organs, namely, in the stomach together with the bowels, and in the system of the skin. When the first organ is diseased and weak, it lacks the ability to convert the consumed aliments, promptly and normally, into chyle and blood; when the second organ is weak and inactive, there is a deficiency in the requisite quantity of blood, because the sluggish skin *does not transpire readily enough* the refuse of the body. When this excretion stagnates, then there is no room and desire for the freshly prepared substance, consequently, no sufficient appetite.

The morbid condition of sluggish digestion is removed by internal use of water; the second one, viz. that of stagnating transpirations, by external use of water. There it is then that the secret lies, why the cold bath increases the appetite so decidedly. If water is not taken internally at the same time, the digestive organs cannot supply as much as the skin excretes, and, consequently, as much as the body requires, without decreasing in weight.

Experience has afforded the average result that, in pursuance of the water-diet, from once and a half to twice as much is eaten, as in pursuance of the old coffee and tea, wine and beer diet; whence the conclusion unquestionably follows, that, under the water régime, the body renews itself from one and a half times to twice as soon as under the old régime. If the natural rotation of the entire renewal of the body embraces four years, it arises to six or eight years with the so-called healthy persons of the old régime; with chronically diseased persons a still longer time, or rather with them there is no radical renovation at all.

The flesh of the body possesses the normal firmness, hardness, and strength only when, according to the appointment of nature, it renews itself rapidly; and, consequently, when the refuse flesh, &c., is rapidly dissolved and transpired; the slower the process proceeds, the more tender, soft, and flabby becomes the flesh, and the organism inclines then, in particular, to the generation of fat, provided that it has no wasting chronic disease. It exceeds the expectation of every one, how a thorough water-cure converts the soft miserable flesh of the coffee, and brandy, and medicine diet into iron-like muscularity.

Heartburn and Eructations, as habitual symptoms, arise from the acidification of the food and drink taken into weak and diseased stomachs, and the endeavor of the stomach to throw them off. The heartburn and eructations are to be viewed as an imperfect effort at vomiting, and it passes over into actual vomiting by the right application of water, whereby the stomach is then cleansed. In most cases this is quickly effected by water, but it requires a much longer time so to heal and strengthen the stomach as to enable it to digest normally, and thus generate no acidity.

Hard and Obstructed Evacuations arise from weakness, inactivity, and from the insufficient secretion of fluid matter in the large intestines, and particularly in the rectum. When the digested chyle is imbibed by the ileum and jejunum, the coarser, and, therefore, not absorbable constituent parts of it remain behind, and pass, drained and desiccated, into the large intestines, into which a considerable quantity of mucous fluid ought to be secreted for the purpose of discharging the excrements. But when the vessels of the bowels are dried up by medicaments and drugging, and partially destroyed; farther, when an inactivity of the rectum is brought on by close sedentary habits, that mucous fluidity is not secreted in sufficient quantity, and thus the evacuations are hard and sluggish.

The Sliming of False Mucus I call that state of disease of the stomach in which the food is not properly decomposed and digested, but turns to a mucus-like mass. This arises in weakness of the stomach, insufficient sharpness and energy of the gastric juice. The usual cause is long-continued use of medicines, whereby the nerves and glands of the stomach have become weakened and partially destroyed.

The Worms of the intestines appear only when disease and slime (false mucus) are present in these organs; they are parasitical animals, which do not exist out of the bowels, and, consequently, never get into the body from without.

The worst variety of these worms is the tape-worm. Many persons take care not to drink water because they are apprehensive of imbibing a young tape-worm; or, at least, one of their eggs. If these persons would only incommode themselves with a little reflection they might easily relieve themselves of such fears. Has any one ever found an old tape-worm in water? No. Whence, then, shall a young tape-worm or an egg of these animals find its way into the water?

A tape-worm may, however, very easily originate in the bowels by total abstinence from water-drinking; for the tape-worm is a parasitical animal, which is generated in weak bowels, and the bowels can only preserve their full energy through the use of cold water.

Whoever uses water with their children internally and externally may rest assured that they will never be tormented with worms and worm-doctors. The expulsion of the small worm by medicine can only have, as a consequence, the generation always of more, because the intestines become weaker and weaker by means of the medicine; strengthen them, and they will cleanse themselves.

The medical mode of expelling the tape-worm is truly horrid. The worm is to be poisoned, or rather, so much poison is to be sent after it that it betakes itself to flight out of sheer fright. A fearful, mad experiment, that has already cost many an one his life, and is quite worthy of allopathy. Must not the poison pass through the stomach, and, consequently, poison the unwilling possessor of the tape-worm either to death or chronic disease? Even when the expulsion of the animal is effected, and the subject escapes with his life, still, the injury which the medicine inflicts upon the bowels is generally much worse than was the burden of the lodgment.

All those causes which produce sliminess and disease of the bowels, may also be the immediate or remote causes of worm disease: medicine, false diet, hot foods and drinks, want of water-drinking, &c.

I remember a tragico-comic occurrence which happened

in my native town; two women, an aunt and her niece, who drank boiled water through fear of drinking in a young tape-worm, and at the same time partook amply of medicine, coffee, and tea; *both* fell a prey to the object of their apprehension.

V.

CONSUMPTIVE DIARRHŒA. THE SLIMING WITH REAL MUCUS. HARDENING OF THE MUCOUS SLIMING, AND INDURATIONS IN THE WALLS OF THE DIGESTIVE CANALS. CHRONIC INFLAMMATION, OR ULCERATION IN THE DIGESTIVE CANALS. CANCER IN THE STOMACH.

THE consumptive diarrhœa results from the total ruin of the absorbing intestines (of the ileum and jejunum). When these intestines do not at all, or very imperfectly, absorb the digested chyle, it passes, with the greater part of its fluid substance, into the large intestines, and is evacuated by them in its liquid state.

Consequently, the secondary or consumptive diarrhœa is the result of processes quite different from those of the primary. While the latter is produced by abnormal secretions of fluid from the large intestines, the former is the result of non-absorption in the small intestines.

It is certain that the consumptive diarrhœa very rarely arises from other causes than continued dosing with strong medicinal poisons; I even believe that it has never arisen from any other cause than poisonings.

The manner in which the coating of the alimentary canal with real mucus is effected, has already been shown in the foregoing. The nature of this disease consists in an abnormally copious secretion of true mucus from the mucous glands. The cause of abnormal secretions of mucus is twofold, as also is the nature of the true mucous slimings.

The first cause is a diseased affection of the mucus-glands, especially a weakness thereof, which is commonly produced by the medical treatment of a primary inflammation of the glands, much more frequently by excessive exertion of individual organs (e. g. the flow of semen, brought on by strong sexual debauches), sometimes, also, by a perverted diet and uncleanliness.

The medicinal poisoning is here, as in every secondary disease, the great chief cause. Under the hands of the physicians, inflammatory, catarrhal, and even intermitting fevers, often enough degenerate into mucous fever. Such a change is possible *only* through poisoning.

This kind of sliming with real mucus, i. e. of abnormal secretions of mucus from disease of the glands, occurs more rarely in the digestive canals.

The second state of true mucous sliming consists in an abnormal secretion of mucus for the purpose of envelopment and dilution of poisonous matters forced upon the organism. This sort of sliming, therefore, does not arise from a disease of the mucus-glands, but from a defensive operation of the organism against inimical substances pressed upon it.

When the digestive organs have become coated with slime, then the old curing art applies medical purgatives to subdue the symptoms.

With a stomach not totally ruined, not uncommonly weak, a vomitive causes the ejection of the food remaining in it, of a part of the vomitive itself, sometimes; also, of the whole of it, also, of the fluids taken into the stomach, and especially of that mucus which has been produced afresh by the poison of the vomitive; in a word, the ejection of all matters free and loose in the stomach. But the original mucous conglomerations of longer standing in the stomach, for the removal of which the emetic was given, and which, by reason of their tenacious viscousness, adhere to the desiccated surface of the walls of the stomach, can never be ejected without being first dissolved and set at liberty. For this purpose the old healing art first administers the so-called resolutive medicines of a decomposing nature. The physicians must have strange notions of the processes going on in the stomach if they suppose these resolutive poisons shall, at command, address themselves to the mucous conglomerations and decompose them. On the contrary, as soon as the new medicine enters the stomach, the stomach must react against it, must prepare fresh mucus in order to envelope it. Instead of dissolving the old phlegm and slime, it always fixes it more firmly than ever, because the stomach is farther exhausted and weakened by every additional poisoning. If an emetic follows the resolutive medicine, there certainly ensues great discharge of slime and bile; *but it is always the mucus and effusion of bile only which have been produced by the medicine just administered,* and, accordingly, are floating loosely in the stomach. The old slime which has been adhering to the walls of the stomach, can be dissolved and removed by nothing else than water.

The case is precisely the same in regard to the purgative medicines, with the difference only, that they cause, particularly in the bowels, fresh productions of mucus, and its partial evacuation.

The oftener such medicinal "purifications" are undertaken, so much the more does the slime accumulate, and if such a course be pursued for a length of time, these medicines finally lose their purgative effect, they accumulate together with the slime in the internal canals—because the reactive power of the organs has been destroyed. At length, the bowels may get completely choked up, and a slow death ensues, which, in excruciating nervous sufferings, cannot be equalled.

If some among my readers are not convinced by what I have already set forth concerning the operation of the medical "means of purification," I can adduce the proof of facts and experience, of such overwhelming force that no resistance is possible; viz. those persons who, having undergone a medical course for the purpose of purifying the stomach, especially for intermitting fever, have come to Graefenberg, have, under the influence of water, obtained a purifying crisis, in which not only great masses of slime have been vomited out, but also the medicine which they had taken, oftentimes plainly recognised by their taste. Those who have been long under medical treatment for stomach complaints, may rest assured that they harbor a great plenty of slime and drug-stuffs in their digestive canals,—may rest assured that, by the water-cure, they will attain a radical purification, if, to wit, they possess sufficient perseverance and the disposition not to break off the cure before or during the crisis.

Perhaps some one, who is not, from his own experience, acquainted with the water-cure, raises the plea here, that the excess of water drinking may excite vomiting and diarrhœa, even when the digestive canals are perfectly clean and sound. Possibly vomiting, but never diarrhœa;

and, moreover, that which is thus vomited is nothing but pure water, free from all nauseous and medicinal taste. This vomiting is only possible when more water is forced into the stomach than it is able to contain by its greatest distension, and the instinct so defends itself against such an act of violence that it never occurs. Circumstances of two kinds prove that old impurities and slime-enveloped medicinal stuffs lie at the foundation of the Graefenberg purification-crises; in vomiting-crises, it is proved by the quantities of slime, and the disgusting taste, which is oftentimes plainly medicinal; in diarrhœa-crises, it is confirmed by the evacuated slime-masses, and an unquestionable proof is the fact that, when the crisis is over, the most energetic water-cure is unable to produce those vomitings and diarrhœas.

The more inconsiderable the coating and sliming of stomach and bowels, the more promptly and easily will the crisis ensue; the more inveterate and accumulated, so much the longer will the crisis be delayed; because, in this case, it requires longer time so to reinvigorate the stomach, &c., that it shall have strength snfficient to produce and carry through the crisis. So soon as the patient feels himself pretty well, and has gained much strength, then the purification-crises commence. Certain it is, that many persons have left Graefenberg without getting the crisis, because they went away too soon, and without misgiving how affairs stood in their bowels.

The circumstances and appearances in persons legitimately poisoned by medicine, have been ascertained to be similar to those in persons illegitimately intentionally poisoned; for instance, in many victims of Gesche Timm. Persons who, according to the confessions made by this insidious murderess before her judges, had received poison from her long before, and died several years after the date of her confessions, had in their stomachs a coating of mucus, which, by chemical examination, was found to contain arsenic. These miserable victims could certainly have been saved by the water-cure timely applied.

In the foregoing we have considered the operation of medicinal emetics upon a stomach not entirely depressed to the lowest degree of weakness. When, however, the stomach is so weak that it is not equal to the strong exertion of the muscles necessary to medical vomiting, and when, consequently, no discharge follows, then it is always certain that the entire medicament remains, during the life-time of the patient, in his body, inasmuch as a small portion of it is received into the digestion; the greater portion of it, however, adheres in mucous slime firmly to the walls of the stomach, after that the stomach has separated the liquid part of the medicament, the original water, from the solid and properly medicinal part. This process it undertakes with every liquid medicament in general; one must not suppose there is any other dripping fluid on our planet excepting water; all other apparently fluids are nothing else than a mixture of infinitely minute solid substances with water. If the chemical arts shall perhaps never be able to resolve completely the intermixed liquids into their original water and original solid atoms, still the stomach can, at least partially, and it effects this partly by its decomposing juice, partly in the case of liquids containing poison by fresh infusions of mucus, which is an excellent filterer, inasmuch as the solid parts remain in it, and the fluid ooze through. The stomach is the best chemist; and the stomach proceeds thus with all mixed liquids which come into it, especially with medicaments always, if it does not discharge them immediately by vomiting or diarrhœa. When, therefore, we speak of medicaments being firmly fixed in the weak stomach, it means only the solid medicinal parts; by no means, however, is it to be presumed that the medicine remains as liquid mixture in the stomach, which, indeed, were manifest nonsense. As soon as the solid parts, the proper quintessence of the medicament, are separated from the watery parts and enveloped in slime in the stomach, then they adhere thereto, and harden to a firm mass, in like manner as the mucus, which, in persons of unhealthy stomach, is generated in the mouth and settles on the teeth, hardens to tartar.

If any one disputes and doubts the correctness of my reasoning concerning the inefficaciousness of medicinal vomitives, viz. that the mucus ejected through such means is only that which is at the time called forth by the same: he may convince himself by administering an emetic to a clean, healthy stomach. So soon as the stomach decomposes it, it feels that it is poison, and that, for a double reason, it must quickly prepare a fresh quantity of mucus; first, to protect itself and its glands, nerves and capillaries, &c., against the poison; second, wherewith to eject it, which cannot be effected otherwise than by the help of this transporting medium; unless great quantities of cold water and milk be drunk immediately upon the emetic, whereby the ability to vomit is guaranteed to the stomach, and the necessity of generating mucus is obviated. If any person, for the sake of gaining a knowledge of the truth in this matter, wishes the experiment made, I would advise him to undertake it under his own supervision, and not commit it to the faith of mediciners, the most of whom disbelieve, entirely, in the efficacy of water as an antidote for poison, and must, from the nature of circumstances, namely, in a struggle on the issue of which depends their own subsistence, and in a time when, alas! truth is not as highly prized as bread.

One might convince himself still more decidedly that emetics call forth mucus in the purest, healthiest stomachs, if he would take, before the emetic, one of those so-called resolutive medicaments, and first allow that to operate an hour.

In a manner quite similar, the medical purgatives cause evacuations of mucus even from the healthiest and cleanest bowels; and in like manner, the evacuations from slime-coated bowels, caused by purgative medicines, never consist of the old morbid matters, but only of fresh-formed mucous-masses.

The course of water-treatment to be pursued in hardened mucous-coatings of the digestive canals, consists in plenteous drinking, in sitz-baths, wet compresses about the body, and clysters; here, as in every other case, we premise, as first postulate of every water-treatment and water-diet, a full cold bath every day.

In cases of old mucous-coatings more water must at first be drunk than the thirst calls for, because the quantum which the thirst requires is soon digested, and, therefore, has no time to dissolve the indurated mucus. Drinking beyond the thirst must never be carried to excess, or it may do injury. A few glasses beyond the thirst suffice to furnish the stomach with the means of solution. As soon, however, as the solution, and in consequence thereof, vomiting or diarrhœa have begun, not a glass must be drunk beyond the thirst.

The sitz-bath, through the coincidence of several effects, is the greatest among the great benefactions wherewith the genius of Priessnitz has favored suffering humanity. The results of this bath, in regard to the re-invigoration of the digestive organs, would appear truly wonderful if they could not be explained on such evidently natural principles.

Firstly, The bath draws long-lodged morbific and medicinal matters out of the external membranes and muscles of the abdomen, inasmuch as it produces there eruptions and boils, and it is particularly efficacious in this respect, on account of the long duration of the bath.

Secondly, It fortifies the nerves of the ganglionic system in a decided manner.

Thirdly, The sitz-bath strengthens as well by the general effect of cold water as, especially, by the wet rubbing and excitation of the abdominal muscles, and promotes the worm-like (peristaltic) motion of the bowels, without which all digestion is impossible.

Fourthly, By its mechanical pressure it promotes vomiting, as soon as it becomes necessary. Other healing effects of the sitz-bath upon other organs belong not here.

The *bandages* assist the sitz-bath in all its operations.

The clysters serve to cleanse and strengthen the rectum, and are a necessary part of the water-cure with all of weak digestion. For wherever there are secretions of slime and weakness of the stomach, there are also sluggishness and accumulation of excrements in the rectum.

Constipation attends not only chronic stomach disease, but, also, almost every acute disease for a time, if it is treated according to the old medicine-régime. This constipation and the medicine quite naturally destroy the appetite, and, indeed, so universally that we are accustomed to view the loss of appetite as a natural and necessary effect of the diseases themselves. Lay hold upon water, ye sick, and you will retain a good appetite and free evacuations, and will perceive that these most important functions are disordered, not by the diseases, but by the medicine alone. In violent fevers under water-treatment the appetite sometimes fails one day, rarely two, and never more.

When a disordered, constipated state of the evacuations has been brought on by medicine during an acute disease, and this function afterwards proceeds again in a normal manner; then, still, the excrementitious matters, whose discharge was delayed days and weeks, remain oftentimes in the rectum, since, by means of slime, they adhere thereto and indurate. The releasement and evacuation of these can be effected only by frequent cold-water clysters; at the same time, the rectum thus regains its former energy. With persons already sunk deep in the miseries of impaired digestion and constipation, the clysters are at first discharged again, before they grow warm in the bowels, and without being followed by the evacuation of much excrementitious matter. One must not allow that to lead him astray, but must continue, and soon the water will be taken up, and whole clysters be entirely absorbed throughout, in proof of the need such bowels have of the healing element. Then normal evacuation ensues, and, after a length of time, perhaps several months, begins the liberation and evacuation of the old filth of the bowels, which has become like unto hard bullets.

As the excrements become very hard and compressed, it is thus possible that the rectum stores away incredibly great quantities in a small space, before it gets so far constipated that atrophy or some other fatal disease ensues. There have been instances at sea where passengers have had no evacuation of the bowels for a long time, even for several weeks, without altogether losing their appetite and health. Of course the abdomen is distended by such accumulations; but still it is astonishing that it can contain the refuse of so many meals. Afterwards, when the usual softer evacuations are again restored without any discharge of the old, hard, dry excrement, then the compass of the abdomen is reduced by their firmer and more compact consolidation, but it never regains its normal symmetry. Despite this internal accumulation, a tolerable state of health may be enjoyed for years; still, if some other disease does not sooner terminate life, it renders a natural death impossible in all cases where chronic disease is harbored in the body.

Those parts of the stomach and bowels which are covered with indurated slime, perish organically, and pass into induration, because these parts are prevented by the slime adhering to them from organic action; they are prevented from secreting digestive juices, and from absorbing chyle; they are prevented from excreting their own refuse, and, therefore, renewal is impossible.

The symptoms of indurated slime in the digestive canals do not manifest themselves unequivocally until the commencement of the water-cure crises, or, after death, in dissections of corpses. The symptoms of disease in all internal indurations and ossifications do not appear well marked in living patients that are not under water-treatment. They are attended with no sensible pains. If the sliming covers only small spaces in the large bowels, no effects are perceptible for a long time, and proper symptoms of the disease sometimes never appear. An internal imperceptible effect is, indeed, always present, and that consists in a somewhat insufficient sustenance of the body. When, however, such like coatings and indurations are present in the stomach, then there are always considerable indurations in the bowels, because, in the latter, especially in the folds of the large bowels, the slime always settles and adheres first. A person is paler and more emaciated in the same ratio that his digestive canals are the more extensively covered with slime and indurations. Accordingly, loss of flesh and paleness of the skin are the chief symptoms of indurated slime, which, when present in a high degree, results in hypochondriasis and painful affections of the nervous system. When a person labors under all these symptoms of disease without having any decidedly marked diseases, then the digestive organs are always the seat of the complaint, and *generally* indurated slime is present in these organs. Persons of solid flesh and ruddy complexion are seldom thus affected, and *never* to any considerable extent.

It is an easy matter to show in what manner the indurated mucous coatings of the stomach and bowels produce emaciation and paleness. According as a greater extent of the surface of these organs is slimed and indurated, so much less surface is in activity in the digestion of food and the absorption of chyle. In this manner a considerable portion of the aliment of the food consumed passes off in excrement, unelaborated and unemployed. For this reason all persons with slime-coated bowels and stomach, are inclined to over-eating, because the body requires more aliment than the digestive organs can elaborate; therefore, despite the large quantity of their daily food, which, with healthy digestion, would be sufficient to the permanent nutrition of a full rugged body, their body continues to emaciate more and more.

Since the great majority of people have not healthy digestive organs, they experience a feeling of great discomfort if they fully satiate their appetite. Hence, then, has arisen the oft-repeated rule, that it is more healthy to cease eating before the appetite is fully satisfied. This precaution is quite necessary for medicine-poisoned stomachs, but for healthy stomachs it is a great folly, if, to wit, an active life be combined with healthiness of stomach. Whoever has his digestion restored by a course of water-cure, and afterwards continues in the diet of Priessnitz, feels himself in the highest degree comfortable and healthy, if he always fully satisfies his appetite; and, indeed, in our temperately cold climate, fat foods are particularly wholesome to the healthy, as well to impart pliancy to the bowels as to maintain a comfortable warmth of body. However, those who have stomachs after the fashion of the old régime, suffer of sour stomach after partaking of fat, and cannot eat it, and dare not, generally speaking, satisfy their appetite; and they also, who lead a sedentary life, should never fully satiate their appetite.

Do you suppose Nature would have given man appetite for more than he dare eat? Do you suppose that Nature would have imposed penances and denials on mankind? No, mankind itself has done it.

When the appetite of the healthy hydropathic stomach is satiated to its utmost requisition with very fat foods, there follows no penance as a consequence thereof, but that satisfactory, in the highest degree pleasurable, condition of digestion which the healthy only know.

Hard and scanty stool is usually connected with sliming of the bowels, and determination of blood to the head, and eyes, and breast. All these consequential disorders and discomforts disappear of themselves as soon as the purification by water is completed. If, instead of which, medicine is still continued in, a sort of consumption sets in also, an iliac passion, a hardening of the intestines, or such like scientifically produced affliction.

The coating and partial induration of the digestive organs is very rarely observed among the lower classes, since there medicinal dosing is not carried to any considerable extent. Nearly all the patients that enter the water-cure establishments have taken a great deal of medicine; according to my experience in establishments *well directed*, and provided with *good water*, about one-half of the patients get critical diarrhœas, and one-eighth part get critical vomiting; consequently, of the cure-guests in water-cure establishments, about one-half bring with them *indurated* sliming of the bowels, and only an eighth part such sliming of the stomach.

From the well-discussed operation of mucous sliming, to which the stomach resorts to protect itself against the poisons forced upon it, we obtain the explanation of the causes why certain doses and kinds of poison introduced into the stomach do not cause immediate symptoms of disease to arise, although, when introduced through a wound into the direct circulation of the blood, they produce speedy death. This is the case with the poison of serpents, of which one may swallow, without perceptible injury, the same quantity which, introduced into a wound, would soon produce either death, or, at least, violent morbid symptoms.

When, however, the doses of poison are too large, and, at the same time, too violent, for the stomach to envelope them through the sliming process, they eat through the slime, and cause, not unfrequently, a chronic ulceration of those places in the stomach and bowels on which they more particularly settle.

Generally speaking, it must be observed under the theme of mixture of poisons with mucus, that an *absolute* envelopment of the poison in mucus is never effected, but only a relative, and that always more or less of the administered poison is absorbed and taken into the circulation; more when the poison mixed with mucus courses through the bowels; less when the greater part thereof remains in the stomach. But yet this latter case is the more pernicious, because the hearth of life, the workshop of the aliment of the body is thus more ruined than when the poison is carried off out of the stomach and partially mixed with the blood.

In a chronic ulceration, the organism, under the usual diet, without assistance from the water-cure, reacts only against the rapid extension of the evil, by constantly conducting its best juices thither to keep in subjection the corroding poison. This imperfect reaction produces that sort of inflammation which the physicians denominate chronic, and which has not an energetic but a sly character. Such reaction allows the ulceration to proceed only very slowly, sometimes retards its progress several years. But as soon as a new debilitating cause, any other disease, or old age arises, the annihilation proceeds more rapidly, and causes death—oftentimes many years after the poisoning has been effected.

The symptoms of this disease are, besides an inadequate digestion and nourishment, a sensation of burning or pricking in the stomach or bowels, which often alternates with a sensation of oppression. In a more advanced state of the disease there ensues, also, vomiting of *coagulated* blood, which escapes from one of the blood-vessels corroded and eaten through by the ulceration or alvine evacuations of blood, which now is coagulated, now not. Generally, periodical vomiting also attends the chronic ulceration of the stomach, still not always.

This disease is cured by water, when sufficient organic strength is still present, and the disease has not yet reached the last stadium. The processes by which water effects cure are easily explained. The water that is drunk makes, as already before observed, its course through the whole circulation of the blood, before it is in part excreted through the urinary organs. It thus releases stagnating and slimy matter, it qualifies acrid and poisonous humors by thinning and diluting them, and conducts them out of the body through transpirations of the skin, and evacuations, and urine, if water be also rightly and proportionably applied externally. In such a manner the water-cure purifies all the juices and the whole mass of the body. Moreover, the water comes in direct contact with the inflamed and festering parts of the digestive canals, and before it enters into the circulation is partially absorbed by these parts in the state of pure water, and mixes itself with the acrid poisonous humors, which are the cause of the inflammation, and thus qualifies and dilutes them, and becomes, at the same time, the medium of their transportation to the place of excretion. In this way it operates from within through the capillaries of the walls of the stomach, and, at the same time, from without the stomach, dissolving, diluting, and extracting. It exercises another healing effect, through its constituent parts, oxygen and hydrogen, in the necessary new formation or reconstruction of nerves, glands, &c., destroyed by the inflammation.

The cancer in the stomach arises from causes similar to those of the chronic inflammation. It is a more obstinate and fatal disease, and is brought on when those causes just mentioned are present in a high degree, particularly when a general and extensive corruption of the humors is combined therewith, and when corrosive and poisonous substances deposit themselves on the glands of the stomach.

The symptoms of cancer in the stomach are the following: first, the concealed symptoms in the stomach, which are only detected by dissection, are, in the beginning, a rough, hard tumor, which is painful, has a red hue, afterwards passing to dark red, to a lead color, and blue-black, which grows into the adjacent parts; finally, bursts and discharges an acrid, oftentimes bloody fluid pus of various colors and offensive odor.

The symptoms of cancer sensible to the patient during life, are, burning and stitching pains in the stomach, vomiting of an offensive watery substance frequently mixed with blood, exceedingly bad digestion, and meagre nourishment of body, sleeplessness, and constipation.

From this, one may perceive that the symptoms of chronic inflammation nearly resemble those of cancer in the stomach.

The cancer is more difficult of cure than the chronic inflammation, but in its commencement, and especially with strong constitutions, it is curable by water. The curative processes are, in every respect, similar to those described in ulceration of the stomach. When, however, the cancer has been open a long time, and the organism extremely emaciated and debilitated in the strife against it, then a cure is no longer possible. I have cured, with water, not a small number of cancer patients; but I have also denied many a reception into my establishment who were already in an advanced stage of this disease, because the hydropath must guard against a case of death in his establishment at almost any price. For this reason he must frequently deny a reception to patients, who are not absolutely incurable, with whom, however, it is *doubtful* whether they may not die before long.

A goodly number of persons bear within them the germ of cancer. These unfortunates in the hands of the drug-doctors journey onward to a horribly painful death. Had they knowledge of their disease, and of the various methods of cure, they would hasten to enter a water-cure establishment before it might be too late. Whoever has a periodical feeling of burning or pricking in the stomach, oftentimes combined with an alternating oppression there, with him the germ of stomach cancer, or, at least, a chronic ulceration, is developing itself.

VI.

MUCUS FEVER. NERVOUS FEVER. PUTRID FEVER.

THE mucus fever arises generally from falsely treated catarrhal and inflammatory fevers, and the false treatment of the latter fevers consists in the employment and administration of medical poisons, and a false diet. To the latter belongs the prohibition of all use of cold water, and using instead thereof warm emollient soups, which are particularly injurious, when the patient manifests an aversion for them, and then still is compelled to take them by order of his physician. It is very rare that a fever sets in immediately with the character of mucus fever.

The symptoms of mucus fever are the following: Quick, but weak pulse, loss of appetite, usually constipation, which sometimes alternates with diarrhœa, pale, also dirty grey color of complexion, tendency to thrush, and the symptoms of foul stomach, eructations from the stomach, coated tongue, a slimy nauseous taste, puffed up abdomen. With these symptoms are combined, oftentimes, catarrhal affections, which in general do not belong to the mucus fever character, but are transferred from their original catarrhal character to the mucus fever.

The cure of the mucus fever is effected through mucous discharges, both of vomiting and alvine evacuations; farther, through critical perspirations, and eruptions. It is evident, from the above given explanations, that all these said curative processes are not only promoted by water, but are brought about by it alone; it is farther evident, that medicinal remedies are decided hindrances to these processes. Under the hands of the doctors, very often a catarrhal fever is converted into mucus fever, and mucus fever into nervous fever ; daily experience teaches it. In the hydriatic treatment, such a change for the worse is an impossibility.

(2.) *The nervous fever* likewise sets in very seldom as the original form of disease, and is as generally as the mucus fever a fabrication of the doctors ; nervous fever developes itself under the doctor's hands from gastric, catarrhal, inflammatory, and even from intermitting fevers. *The nervous fever* is not a healing disease ; what I have said in my first hydriatic work, entitled, " The Spirit of the Graefenberg Water-Cure," upon this fever, proceeded from a wrong view of this disease, and requires the rectification here given. That pamphlet was written by me during the first period of my own water-cure, and wants the eight years' experience and investigations, which since that time I have collected and prepared.

The nervous fever arises, when an organism, afflicted with morbific matters, receives an impulse to the production of a healing fever ; *at the same time, however, the weakness of the nerves, and also usually the relaxation of the system of the skin, steps in the way, hindering the accomplishment of a healing form of disease.* Under healing fevers, I include the inflammatory, catarrhal, gastric, and intermitting fevers.

From this explanation concerning the nature of nervous fever, we get also an explanation of the causes, why the said healing fevers, under the hands of the doctors, so often degenerate into nervous fevers, to wit, because by blood-letting and poisonings the organism is robbed of the power necessary to maintain and perfect the healing fever ; because the nervous system is depressed by these disturbing inroads, and thereby disqualified for any healing fever, and, finally, because from non-application of water to the skin, that system in all fevers and sweatings is so depressed, that critical discharges therefrom cannot possibly ensue in a satisfactory manner. Under all these hindrances the excitation then passes over to the nervous system in particular; *nervous afflictions and violent fever combine to form a compound disease, which is denominated nervous fever.*

It has already been shown in the foregoing, that the gastric fevers frequently have an epidemic cause, i. e. they originate in a corruption of the air in certain districts. These gastric fevers of the epidemic nature are, under the hands of mediciners, very frequently converted into nervous fevers; indeed, in certain districts, and at certain times, they *always* assume, without delay, the nervous form under drug treatment. Therefore it is quite an error to speak of epidemic or contagious nervous fevers; for, in the water-treatment, the gastric fevers never assume the marked nervous form, and they soon lose those symptoms which prognosticate a degeneration of the fever into the nervous form.

In consideration of the causes of nervous fever it should not remain unmentioned, that, when a disposition of the body to arouse a healing fever is present, mental over-exertion may likewise become a cause of degeneration into nervous fever. Farther, this disease may develope itself from a healing fever, by means of repeated deleterious mental excitements, through fright, great fear, grief, and repeated vexations. But all these causes occur very seldom, in comparison with the causes of bloodletting and medicinal poisoning; for those mental and moral causes must rise to an unusually fearful degree, if they are to produce an effect equal to the medical treatment.

The symptoms of nervous fever are the following : Every kind of nervous fever is ushered in by disturbances in the head, nervous pains, feverish pulse, loss of appetite, and sleep, or at least the sleep is unrefreshing, and beset with fantasies. Nervous fever is divided into two general kinds.

(1) The inflammatory nervous fever approaches more nearly the curative form of disease than the torpid nervous fever, and the former is more easily and certainly curable by water than the latter. In the inflammatory nervous fever we perceive a greater energy in all the functions of the organism, and in all manifestations of disease. Dry, and burning hot skin, rapid and irregular pulse, state of high excitement and deliriousness, parching thirst, nervous, and sometimes half rheumatic pains, dry, brown, cracked tongue ; these constitute the most prominent symptoms of inflammatory nervous fever.

(2) The torpid nervous fever has on the other hand the following symptoms ; pale and sunken expression of countenance, lack-lustre, dying expression of the eye, total prostration of the strength, dulness of the senses, in contradistinction to the diseased sensitiveness of the senses in the inflammatory nervous fever, torpid slumbering, entire want of appetite and of evacuations from the bowels, dark brown furrowed tongue, gloomy unconscious fantasies.

The inflammatory nervous fever is very often converted into the torpid by medical treatment. The further effects of that treatment are either death, through palsy, apoplexy, exhaustion of the vital energies, resolution of the juices of the body, consumption of the nerves (suppressed nervous fever), or a very slow and relative recovery, without any or at least any considerable struggles and discharges. How tardily convalescence follows, under medical hands, and how very seldom the former state of health is afterwards regained, are circumstances sufficiently well known, and find their most satisfactory explanation herein, viz. that the critical discharges of the morbific matter are rendered impossible by medical treatment.

In the hydriatic treatment, nervous fever assumes, gradually, the character of rheumatic or catarrhal fever; also, marked rheumatic pains usually arise, and the matters of disease, which have occasioned the nervous fever, are eliminated through critical secretions. If the disease be treated *from the very commencement* with water, its radical cure is effected very soon, comparatively, and after-pains, relapses, or, indeed, the origination of new chronic affections, are never consequent upon such treatment.

Although the hydriatic treatment of nervous fever must be more carefully undertaken than that of inflammatory fevers, and although the nervous fever is a secondary disease, and caused by hindrance being offered to the healing propensity of nature; still, my experience and knowledge have justified me in the belief that no person can die of nervous fever if, in the beginning, it be treated rightly (not after the manner of the physicians), with water. During the prevailing disposition in Mecklenburg for many years past to nervous fevers, I have had occasion to treat this disease in all its stadia and in all its varieties. Although I have never lost a patient by it, not even in cases where a medical treatment had preceded mine, still, I consider the issue of the water-treatment very doubtful when a mediciner has already been previously practising upon the fever. For in so dangerous a disease one does not change from one method of cure to another out of mere pastime, ; one does not discharge his medicine-doctor before that he has abandoned all hope of a fortunate issue of the disease under the medical treatment, and then the patients are already to the last degree emaciated and debilitated. All those that have been handed over to me from the medical treatment, were already reduced to the appearance of skeletons, and I consider it to be, therefore, only a fortunate circumstance that I have also cured all these. Yet, abstractly of the uncertain issue of the water-cure after preceding medicinal treatment, the recovery after such a preceding treatment *is always tedious.*

(3) *The Putrid Fever* is still more decidedly than the nervous fever, a fabrication from primary fevers, and, consequently, seldom comes on immediately in its terrible form. Medical treatment, and a hot, damp, and corrupted atmosphere, are the usual causes, which convert a primary or a nervous fever into a putrid fever.

The Symptoms of Putrid Fever are a pricking heat, which, on being touched with the hand, leaves behind a disagreeable sensation, great debilitation, and disfigured look, a *small* fever-pulse, offensive evacuations, and discharges of blood, *an inclination towards resolution of the humors, and dissolution of the solid parts.*

Although I cannot assert that water, rightly applied, will, *in every case,* cure the putrid fever, yet it is proved, by experience, that water is the best remedy for this disease also, and that one may presume upon a happy issue with great probability, if it be applied immediately in the commencement of this terrible disease.

VII.

NERVOUS AFFLICTIONS. CRAMPS.

ALL nervous afflictions are secondary manifestations of disease, and for this reason their symptoms are not to be considered as healing endeavors of the organism, but are tormenting sensations which the body suffers in its gradual annihilation by chronic disease.

Protracted and lingering nervous afflictions are, in most cases, an effect of secondary disease of the digestive organs, whose disease may be so latent that one detects no symptoms of disease in those parts of the body which are influenced by these organs. For instance, the indurated mucous sliming of the digestive canals has no symptoms particularly sensible in the stomach and bowels, not even when it is present in a very high degree : the signs of the disease are emaciation, paleness, hypochondria, disgust of life : in a word, dull nervous distress, respecting whose true seat the feelings give no proper direction.

The nerves are mostly governed and influenced by the brain ; but the brain itself is a complication of nerves, and if we do not separate it from the nerves of the rest of the body, but place it under the nervous system collectively, then the digestive organ is, of all other organs, that one which exercises the most influence upon the whole nervous system ; the stomach, by means of its ganglionic nerves, stands in reciprocal action with the whole nervous system ; still, however, it influences the nervous system in a higher degree than it is influenced by it.

Since the administered poisons arrive first in the stomach and bowels, before they pass into the blood, and since they are often partially withheld from passing into the blood and the rest part of the body, they being enveloped in mucus, and thus remain in the digestive canals: therefore, among such nations as have, for a long course of time, made use of a method of curing diseases by poisons, the great body of diseases of the digestive organs must not only be widely extended, but, also, preponderate over the diseases of the other organs. Since, farthermore, the digestive organs exercise so decided an influence on the nerves, therefore, nervous afflictions must, next in order, be the most widely extended.

Thus it is in present Europe—everywhere stomach disease, partly in forms of diseases which, by sensual perceptions, denote the stomach as the seat of affliction, partly in latent forms, which manifest themselves to the perception in the form of nervous afflictions.

As the use of medicine among the higher classes is more frequent than among the lower, therefore, with the former, stomach and nervous diseases must be more frequent than among the latter. Experience also confirms this conclusion.

Every poisoning, which causes slow death, not only the medical, but also that of the insidious villain, is followed by a train of dreadful nervous torments.

When the stomach, and especially the ganglionic nerves, are strongly poisoned and shattered by *powerful* medicinal poisons administered in an energetic acute disease, or when some other organ is similarly affected by absorption of the poison from the blood, and when nervous complaints are in such wise produced, then the physicians prescribe *milder* poisons for the cure of these complaints, and thereby complete, slowly but surely, the ruin of the nerves.

These milder poisons are called nerve-strengthening ("neurotic"), or also, in general, "restoratives."

An organism can only be truly restored and strengthened by expelling all foreign matters, especially from the digestive canals, and enabling it to digest and assimilate to itself a sufficient quantity of aliment. This true invigoration is *always* (the water-cure has proved it a thousand times), with very emaciated persons, accompanied by a very sensible, oftentimes astonishing, increase in flesh and muscle, and with persons of sufficient, but soft, weak flesh, it hardens itself to an iron-like solidity. Wherever both of these very visible effects, and, moreover, a blooming ruddy complexion, fail, their true invigoration has never been effected, but at most a false show of it, caused by stimulants. Alcohol is the real main principle of most allopathic "restoratives" or "tonics," which at first spur up the nerves temporarily, in order afterwards to ruin them and the whole organism more surely. The alcohol is then administered, sometimes alone in sublimated form, in ethers, essences, drops, sometimes together with other stimulants; for instance, old wine, cognac, with china, &c. All these articles correspond, in their substance and effects, with brandy. When the period of their first stimulation is past, then bluntness and insensibility follow, and that dreadful condition in which the brandy and stimulants have become a necessity, without being longer able to exercise any effect.

But the etherial lady abstains from brandy as little as the day laborer, when, in her delicacy, she entitles it—ether, eau—and who knows with what other names?

The completion of the ruin of the nerves by nerve-strengthening and narcotic medicaments, rests upon a *direct* pernicious effect of these stuffs on the nerves. Every other poisoning, which produces long-continuing and oft-returning pains, operates, also, *indirectly*, with destructive effect upon the nerves. Pain is a thing which is unnatural, and the nervous system of all animals is constituted for their pleasure, and not for their pain; for this reason it cannot endure long-continuing pain without becoming diseased. Also, rheumatic pains, viz. those of the teeth and of the face, ruin the nerves in the course of time; even the pains produced by external artificial means, e. g. by the tortures of the rack, effect the same, if they are frequently repeated.

When powerful medicinal poisons penetrate directly into the body of the nerves, by means of the circulation, they effect not only a chemical transformation of the substance of the nerves, but also an organic deformation, and respective destruction of the form of the nerves. When, however, medicinal poisons ruin the nervous system through indirect effect, then the transformations usually extend more to the form, than to the material, of the nerves.

The artificial stimulants, which are such dangerous enemies to the nerves, come not alone from the hands of the mediciners, but at the present day, also, out of the lap of the false conditions of culture, particularly from the corruption of social culture. This deep corruption has advanced, indeed, to that degree that the use of narcotic poisons passes for an attribute of manhood, with boys even, as the dub of knighthood, which elevates them to men. Tobacco and the intoxicating drinks belong most particularly to the narcotic poisons. On this point I will here only state, in general, that these pernicious substances are, indeed, much less injurious than the most nerve-poisoning medicaments, but still they are, by all means, injurious to the stomach and nerves, and if they, *of themselves alone*, do not possess the power, when used moderately, *to cause speedy and marked* injury to a healthy person, still they are faithful allies to the medicinal poisons in the work of destruction of the nerves. In the second part I will speak at large respecting tobacco and alcohol.

Also, coffee, tea, and the stimulating spices, are prejudicial to the health of the nerves, although they, of themselves alone, are still less capable than tobacco and alcohol, of destroying a healthy nervous system. But they are co-operative with the destroying power of medicinal poisons, and they must be unconditionally prohibited in all cases where the nerves are already the prey to disease, or a cure will be rendered impossible.

We will now turn to the immaterial causes of nervous affliction. If such causes, without the introduction of foreign matter into the body, can produce disease and gradual ruination to a system of the body, it is unquestionably the nervous system. Still, I do not believe that a case has ever yet occurred in which this system has become diseased through immaterial causes *alone;* but unquestionably these causes are sometimes the predominating, and very often the co-operating causes of disease of the nerves.

First in order, among the immaterial causes as destroyers of the nerves, stand the over-exercise and too close application of the mental faculties. In my opinion there is only one kind of exercise of mind, which is no detriment to the health, and that is the exercise of the ingenuity in enabling us to escape dangers, to pursue enemies and beasts of prey, as this so often occurs in the life of the savages. But abstract and scientific thinking I hold to be relatively unhealthy, and am of the opinion, that at this moment while I am thinking and writing for the interests of the general health, I am acting against the interests of my own health. I say "relatively" unhealthy, and intend by this word to note especially the consideration that it is unnatural and unhealthy to practise abstract thinking as a business and means of livelihood; according to my opinion, every person in a truly human, refined, and cultivated state of society, should busy himself with *some* bodily labor, and the mentally endowed should, only in their hours of recreation, yield themselves up to abstract and scientific thinking as a means of pleasure. That would be not only better for health, but unspeakably much better for science also. Sciences constructed by persons that are recluses by profession, can be as little healthy as are the recluses themselves. But that belongs not here; that digresses widely into strange fields; that draws down much affliction upon humanity, and the poor wan journeyman of science; that gives testimony to the falseness of our refined conditions, and causes me bitter sorrow whenever I reflect upon it; therefore, for four important reasons I must abandon these thoughts.

I said "relatively," and intend thereby to denote the disproportionately constant thinking to the neglect of the corporal elaboration of one's organic powers and his stagnating juices. Every mental occupation that is not pursued from inclination, or choice, or with aversion even, operates either in blunting or morbidly exciting the nerves of the brain, and in every case causes decided injury not to the body only, but also to the mind.

To the over-exertion of the mind belong also the labors of those unhappy writers and poets, whose imagination is not a fountain gushing spontaneously from the lap of the soul, profuse and unceasing, but a pump, which is wrought in the bitter sweat of hard laboriousness.

The second class of immaterial causes of nervous diseases consists of mental affections of an uninjurious kind. To these belong grief, care, fright, and long-continued fear, anger, envy, and jealousy ; also, humbled pride and inordinate thirst after honor and power. All these influences are co-operative with the causes of nervous diseases ; it may be easily supposed that some of these may become causes of nervous afflictions, although this has, by no means, been demonstrated, and experience seems to speak to the contrary. For experience teaches that, of all the above-mentioned mental affections, there is no one which, in every case, will ruin the nervous system of the person therewith affected ; but experience teaches that every lingering poisoning, that of the insidious murderer, as well as of the mediciner, brings wretched disease upon the nervous system ; experience teaches that those persons who have taken the most medicine always have the most diseased nerves.

Sexual excesses also operate injuriously upon the nervous system, but only then, when at the same time a diet of narcotic artificial stimulants is employed, or when medicinal poisoning is present. If a natural diet is used, and the water-cure employed when the disease occurs, then with healthy persons of mature age, there can be no excesses, in as far as *health* is concerned, i. e. the inclination to physical love does not then exceed the capability thereto.

But quite otherwise is it with sexual pleasures in unripe age, and with all unnatural modes of quieting the sexual desire. They all exhaust the vital energy prematurely, and depress all the mental and corporal functions ; therefore, they depress, also, the nervous system, and rob it of its fresh susceptibility for enjoyment ; but if neither medicinal poisoning, nor mental and moral affections of an injurious nature, nor as yet the pernicious effects of a narcotic diet, co-operate, at the same time, to enhance the evil, then they destroy the whole machine gradually, without producing either symptoms of disease or a strongly prominent disorder in the balance of the functions. Still it is very rare that the said excesses are left to operate alone, as in the supposed case ; when, however, they are attended by a narcotic diet, it assists in annihilating the nervous system.

Cramps are forms of disease which only appear when the nerves are secondarily and deeply diseased. Cramps are involuntary movements and convulsions of the nerves, which impart themselves, more or less, to the adjacent muscles, and through them produce the most various, involuntary, and ungovernable actions of the organism, tossing of the arms and legs, utterance of tones which are now lower, now louder, but always of a fearful kind, and which sometimes swell to a heart-rending shriek.

The allopathic classifications of cramps in clonic, atonic, convulsive, cataleptic, epileptic, &c., are a confused mixture of several modes of classification, because some are only different grades in the effects of similar causes ; others, however, the effects of dissimilar causes.

Next to the organic devastations and deformations, the chronic nervous afflictions are those diseases for which water affords the slowest and most imperfect aid; still, water is, of all remedies, that one which decidedly is capable of affording the greatest relative assistance, and, indeed, the only assistance. This most physicians themselves admit; many of these physicians tell their patients that water is a suitable remedy for nervous affections *only*, well knowing that it cures them the most slowly and imperfectly; often these sly foxes find, among the public, persons who are simple enough to receive such like untruths in good faith.

In regard to the water-cure practically, the chief fundamental rule to be observed in the treatment of severe nervous complaints is, that cold water must never be used until considerable improvement has taken place, but until such time, tepid water of a temperature between 57° and 75° Fahrenheit. This fundamental rule, I am sorry to say, is daily disregarded in many water-cure establishments. By the use of too cold water and too stimulating baths, the condition of the nervous patient is in every case much aggravated, and he may, by such treatment, even be brought into a state of insanity.

During the several past generations of man the acute diseases have become more seldom, and the chronic conditions of disease more frequent (a necessary effect of the medicinal art), and, therefore, the *stimulating medicines* have grown more and more in general use, and the ruin of the nerves and cramps more aggravated. Nervous complaint, over-stimulation of the nerves, cramps, and convulsions, we now find everywhere: in men's bodies, in society, in literature, politics, and morals, and the prime cause of all this evil is nothing else than medicinal poisoning.

Thus allopathy has penetrated with her infernal influences even into the profound depths of the mind. Do you smile? Do you believe, then, that the over-stimulated, nervous weakling can produce thoughts, ideas, deeds, upon which the stamp of disease and nervous over-stimulation is not fixed? Youth is inexhaustible in the talent of hope; it holds the cramps and twinges of our time, for pains of that time, which will give birth to a new grand epoch. Poor deluded youth, the cramps of an over-stimulated poisoned dame are no pains of travail; they are the slow pains of death!

VIII.

HYPOCHONDRIACISM AND HYSTERIA. DISGUST OF LIFE AND SUICIDAL PROPENSITY.

Hypochondriacism and Hysteria are forms of disease similar to one another, and whatsoever is dissimilar in them arises from the dissimilarity of the two sexes; hypochondriacism appertains to the male, and hysteria to the female sex. The seat of both diseases is in the stomach and bowels, and particularly in the nerves. In hysteria, disease of the sexual nerves is always combined with disease of the nerves of the digestive organs; in hypochondria, however, there is usually disease only of the latter nerves present.

The symptoms of the two forms of disease, which they have in common with each other, are, at first, frequent and sudden changes of humor, and, accordingly, apparent changeableness of character. Now unrestrained joy from trifling causes, and again, and still oftener the deepest concern and disquietude, ill temper, vexation, sudden bursts of passion over the most unimportant matters. In the first disposition of temperament, the character appears pleasing, sympathizing, and forbearing; in the second, on the contrary, it appears rough, harsh, unjust, even malicious. A second symptom of these two diseases is selfishness, accompanied, also, with the passion of speaking much of one's own self, and one's own disease, and of reading, meditating, and speculating much upon it, of daily changing one's view with respect to it, and, in imagination, living to experience all possible diseases. With the described eccentricity in each of the most diverse temperaments, they are, of course, also connected with a want of perseverance in any one undertaking, and a seizing after new projects.

In hysteria there is often an unmistakable effort to excite attention by actions, by talking, looks, and in particular, also, by dress, and this propensity appears to arise from disease of the sexual nerves.

The purely corporal symptoms of diseases are pains and cramps in the stomach and bowels, hard and scanty evacuations, flatulency, changeableness in appetite, and a feeling of bodily anxiety and fear. In the hysteria the cramps increase sometimes to convulsions, and to a cramp-like action from abdomen to stomach and throat. It must, however, be observed that the corporal symptoms of disease here enumerated do not always arise, at least, it frequently is the case, that for a long time the above-mentioned conditions of the temperament only show themselves.

The causes which produce hypochondria and hysteria are over-excitement, disorganization, material and formal alteration of the abdominal nerves, effected particularly by oft-repeated purgatives; farther, want of bodily exercise, much sitting, connected with over-exercise of mind, a diet weakening to the digestive organs through overstimulation, sometimes, also, sexual excesses, particularly unnatural sexual indulgences.

In all secondary stomach diseases, therefore, also, in hysteria and hypochondria, the feelings of the patient afford him no sure key to the seat of the disease. The cause of this circumstance lies in the following construction of the human body: the nerves of the abdominal viscera form a separate system, whose centre is called the abdominal brain (cerebrum abdominale). These bowels, as also the heart, receive their nerves from the ganglions, by which the conduct upwards to the head is arrested. Through this isolation from the brain, follows, necessarily, that the said bowels can only transmit their sensations very imperfectly to the brain; moreover, their sense of feeling is, of itself, very weak, because these nerves contain but little marrow.

Most physicians attribute these diseases to dynamic causes; still, many acknowledge, that organic defects and deformations are present in the abdominal organs in these forms of disease, but indeed without comprehending that these disorganizations are rarely produced otherwise than by medicinal poisonings.

They consist in transformation of the material of the nerves, in destruction and induration of the nerves in places, by adhesions of indurated slime, in accumulations of serous fluid (abdominal dropsy), in causing abnormal growths of mucous membrane (polypi), and in chronic ulcerations.

The hypochondria and hysteria are always real diseases of the body; the supposition that these complaints sometimes originate in the imagination merely, is utterly false. Of the seat and nature of his disease, the hypochondriac has frequently very erroneous notions; but in regard to the presence of disease he is never deceived. Universally, every one who feels himself unwell, is, in reality, unwell, although the medical advisers often try to reason their patients out of this idea, and persuade them that the disease has been destroyed by their medicines. On the other hand, many consider themselves at times healthy, who are not so, if we assume organic simplicity of body as a condition of true and perfect healthiness.

Hypochondria and hysteria are attended always with periods of despair and disgust of life; still, habitual disgust of life is no symptom of genuine hypochondria, but it springs from a form of disease which is compounded of hypochondria, of sensual surfeiting, and a tough and thick quality of the blood and of the humors. This diseased quality of blood arises from insufficient use of water, and instead thereof the use of fermented and distilled drinks. Under such diet the fluids of the body lack the normal quantity of oxygen and hydrogen, and this want causes an uncomfortable, pleasure-killing feeling in the whole sensorium of the organism; moreover, this want causes a predisposition to apoplexy and such like diseases.

The hypochondriacal, periodical, and habitual disgust of life is, at the present day, so widely extended, and, in itself, brought to such a perfect form, that it may almost be considered as a new temperament. Its chief, or at least, a co-operating cause, lies in the ruin of the digestive organs, as in general all different temperaments are, principally, the results of a healthy or diseased digestion. This has been proved, very conclusively, by the water-cure, which, by restoring to health this important organ, has already metamorphosed many a melancholic malcontent temperament into a joyous, happy, sanguine temperament.

Against these said evils the water-cure is the only remedy capable of effecting anything; it effects, in most cases, where the patient has sufficient perseverance, a radical cure, which, however, for its permanency, requires a reasonable corresponding diet, and particularly that bodily exercise be not neglected. But the water can, of course, not cure when the vital energy is already much exhausted, and those above-mentioned organic defects and ravages in stomach and bowels are, in high degree, advanced.

The highest degree of hypochondria and disgust of life is the suicidal propensity. It is very difficult, it is almost impossible, that a perfectly healthy man raise the armed hand against his own life, although the severest outward disappointments of life almost overcome him. All this outward unhappiness is nothing in comparison to the inward chronic misery of disease.

It is said the passions drive men to commit suicide. Most assuredly; well observed, however, the passions are, in most cases, and with most men, the offspring of disease of body. The perfectly healthy person has rarely and but few passions, because his claims upon the enjoyment of life are satisfied through the pleasures of good digestion and procreative powers. Does some one accuse me of making man half a beast? Not I, but Nature has done it, when she clothed the soul in the garb of an animal body, and—let him also declaim against it who will—still, it is certain that no human soul can be healthy when the shackles of the outward animal, into which it is exiled, are afflicted with pains and wretchedness.

The thirst after happiness speeds through the heart of man powerfully and ardently as the gulf-stream through the ocean. The honey of joy flows in upon the healthy person from all sides; when he awakes in the morning he is full of joy at the prospect of a new day, and with him his limbs, which, refreshed, unfold themselves from the embraces of sleep; he finds joy and refreshment in his very breath, which, with expanded lungs, he inhales from the grand bowl of ether; he reaps delight in viewing the golden sunshine and the streams of the mountains. But with the loss of health flies also the capability of enjoyment and rejoicing, and still the ardent desire for happiness remains. It is a fundamental trait in the perverted condition of the diseased, that they suppose they lack the external conditions of joy, while, indeed, they lack only the internal. Permanent happiness dwells only in the natural enjoyments of a healthy body and mind; when disease dispels these, the wretch longs after strange artificial enjoyments, and the more these escape his grasping hands, the more ardently glows the passion. When the power to love is poisoned by disease, then comes the passion for wealth, and power, and honor, orders and titles, and other insignificancies.

Since most passions are the offspring of disease, the

apparent wonder that water cures them, easily explains itself—because it cures the cause of them.

I am aware that this view sounds quite matter-of-fact-like, is not poetical; the water-cure is not at all so; also, that is not at all requisite to poesy, least of all, to this modern poesy, which puts out its blossoms from a diseased stock. Laugh, laugh, still I fear not to say, make the human race healthy, and you will behold a new poesy arise, the rents and chasms will disappear, the accords of melancholy and shrills of despair cease to resound.

Never has a man in acute disease, during the severest pains and extremities, taken his own life, because instinct feels that they are nothing else than the curative processes of nature. On the contrary, in chronic disease, the feeling of despair awakes, and whispers despondency. Thus the most suicides are the after-consequences of medicinal poisoning, are explosions of the dull feeling of an internal misery, that can be cured by no other pills except the leaden.

Despite the external wretchedness that weighs upon the lower orders, still suicides among them are more seldom, in proportion, than among the higher of society. Their poverty, which allows them to buy but little medicine, protects them against suicide and nervous misery.*

Behold the different men, and observe what different courses they pursue when overtaken by equal strokes of outward misfortune. A bankruptcy drives one to commit

* In more recent times most afflictions among the lower classes are the effect of the poison contained in brandy, viz. alcohol, which corresponding afflictions in the higher classes are produced by medicinal poisoning. Namely, the suicides and shatterings of understanding are among the consequences of the brandy-plague.

suicide, the other, to increased industry, to contentment and true happiness. The faithlessness of a sweetheart breaks the heart of one and sends a bullet through his brain; the other finds another, and becomes the happy head of a family. Whence the different effects of the same causes? From the different temperaments of men, i. e. from the different states of health of their digestive organs.

IX.

RHEUMATISM.

RHEUMATISM falls into several subdivisions, of which the acute or inflammatory rheumatism is properly the only purely rheumatic original form; the cold chronic and the atonic are secondary forms, which are only produced by false treatment of the acute rheumatism. The nervous rheumatism is a compound form of nervous and rheumatic affection.

The Symptoms of Inflammatory Rheumatism are a violent pain, attended with abnormal accumulations of blood, and thereby produced abnormal heat in the affected part. It will be seen that these symptoms are nearly related to the symptoms of the proper inflammatory diseases, and, also, the nature of the two kinds of diseases is similar.

The difference lies herein, that in the inflammatory diseases, the heat and accumulation of blood in the diseased part are greater than in the rheumatic form of disease; also, that the purely inflammatory form runs its course and comes to some decision sooner than the rheumatic; on the other hand, in the rheumatic form the pains are more sensible than in the inflammatory; and finally, this inflammatory form is attended with stronger fevers than the rheumatic. These differences arise partly from the higher energy of the inflammatory form of disease, partly from the essential difference in the organs, which are most frequently attacked by both of the said forms. Thus the internal fleshy organs, and those most abundantly provided with veins, are most subjected to inflammations, while on the other hand, the seat of rheumatism is more in the muscles, membranes, and sinews of the flesh surrounding the bones. Hence, the more sensible pain of the rheumatic, as, also, the more violent accumulation of blood and heat of the inflammatory form explains itself.

From the foregoing it is apparent that the rheumatism is a transition form between the healing and destroying diseases.

The rheumatic pain is caused thereby that the nerves in the affected parts of the body come in contact with foreign acrid substances, particularly with poisonous medicinal substances. Every considerable poisoning with mercury produces rheumatic or gouty pains, which are frequently of exceeding violence.

If one applies acrid corrosive substances externally to the nerves of a wounded part, there arise, quite in the same manner as with the internal rheumatic, inflammatory, and gouty processes, pains, which are the more violent the more corrosive the poisonous substance.

The effect of the water-treatment of inflammatory rheumatism is the expulsion of the matters producing them, through critical sweats and critical exanthems (boils and eruptions).

The effect of the medical treatment is, on the contrary, the conversion of inflammatory rheumatism to cold-chronic, atonic, and nervous rheumatism. This change is thus brought about slowly but surely, that the organism is weakened by medicinal sudorifics, by purgatives, vesicatories, and the like, and prevented from the formation of healing exanthems; farthermore, thus, that the skin of the affected parts is long covered with flannel and oiled silk, and thereby totally weakened and rendered absolutely incapable of excreting the morbific matters.

The medicinal sudorifics produce like process with the medicinal purgatives only in other organs. An elimination of morbific matters by the introduction of fresh evil substances is not possible; in the most fortunate, but very rare, cases, the organism succeeds in excreting the newly introduced medicinal evil matters. The sweating caused by medicinal remedies is not a critical perspiration but the sweat of agony; moreover, the stomach is debilitated, and, in the long run, entirely ruined by these remedies usually administered very hot. People say, in common life, the causes of rheumatic affections lie mostly in colds. I have already before shown that no disease and no pains can be produced by the severest cold, if no morbific matters are present in the body. Consequently, a cold, when morbific matters are present in the body, may very well be the incidental cause of exciting rheumatism, and hastening the period of its outbreak, but never can it be the prime cause of it, never produce it.

The chronic cold rheumatism manifests itself only through inward pain, without the skin becoming reddened or heated, because the skin-system and the whole organism is too much weakened to drive the healing signs of heat and accumulation of blood to the periphery.

The atonic rheumatism shows itself in weakness, lameness, and stiffness of the affected parts, without pain and without inflammation.

The nervous rheumatism is that form which the rheumatism assumes with persons of shattered nerves; then convulsive sensations are combined with the rheumatic pains.

The chronic, atonic, and nervous rheumatism cannot, even with the best diet, be cured by the organic strength without the aid of water; still less is this possible by medicinal means. When the water-cure is used properly and with perseverance, and vital energy is still present, then these rheumatic secondary forms are transformed into the primary or inflammatory, which then discharge their morbific humors in critical sweatings and exanthems.

Sometimes the rheumatism remains for a long time settled in one spot, and is then called *the fixed;* sometimes the rheumatic pain flies from one place to another, and is then called the vagrant or unfixed. The vagrant rheumatism is not so to be understood, as if the acrid matters, which generate the pains, changed quickly their position from one place to another, which is a physiological impossibility, but rather in this manner, that the foreign matters are present in different parts of the body, and are set free out of the mucous envelopment in one part of the body by the afore-described processes, and by their acridness produce the pains; these, however, on not being discharged by the excretory functions, are again enveloped in newly infused mucus, whereupon they are set free in other parts of the body and thus generate fresh pains.

When the rheumatism attacks the organs of sense and is medically treated, they are frequently rendered incapable of performing their offices; in such a manner has many a person lost his hearing, his sight, his sense of smell, and not unfrequently even his organ of taste. On the other hand, these diseases of lost senses have been often cured again by water-treatment.

The worst kinds of the fixed rheumatism are lumbago and pains in the face; still these complaints are generally of a complex nature, and have gouty and nervous admixtures. Also, these complaints, the vital energy being sufficient, are cured by water.

One of the most widely-extended and painful rheumatic complaints is the toothache.

Of all those who incessantly feed from the drug-shop, there are very few, perhaps none at all, who are not at times subject to the torments of toothache. Still, the high-seasoned foods and those prepared with sharp acids, bring into the body substances which, by their contact, cause pain in the nerves, and particularly in the nerves of the teeth.

Most medicaments commence their destructions first in the mouth, throat, and the digestive canals, because they are taken most directly in these parts, and, therefore, they penetrate them the most. Before the medicine reaches the stomach, a part of it is absorbed in the tongue, in the gums, in the glands; to be sure the organism reacts against it and endeavors to secrete it in an increased flow of saliva; however, when the use of it is bravely followed up, the power of reaction becomes less and less, and chronic accumulations are deposited. When now a cold is contracted, these minute atoms of poison are loosed from their envelopment, and by reason of their corrosive nature excite pains in the teeth and glands, &c.

As long as the organism is still vigorous, it endeavors to expel the excited matters, through salivation and smaller and larger gum-boils.

The acrid salivation is never anything else than the effect of a new or old poisoning, most frequently caused by mercury; as that same abominable poison, which is now administered for almost every disease, is also the most frequent cause of toothache. Through the salivation somewhat of the penetrating poison is again eliminated; it is unquestionably certain that particles of poison are contained in the acrid saliva; for it could not, possibly, for instance, smell of mercury if there was no mercury in it. Although the physicians must know this, for they know that the sensation of smell is awakened only by material particles coming in contact with the olfactory nerves; they know, also, that the salivation or flow of saliva, though its acridity, corrodes to soreness the lips and mouth—still, these gentlemen seem not to comprehend that the salivation is, therefore, a healing effect of the body, and, consequently, must be supported, which, indeed, is possible only by water. Aye, most physicians give even medicines to suppress the salivation, and for this purpose order piquant, biting substances and spices to be chewed, or give sulphur and iodine, especially in mercurial salivation. Take water in the mouth, and hold it therein until it becomes warm, lay about the throat and saliva glands warming cold-water compresses, bathe daily, and you will see how the secretion of the poison is promoted through increased flow of saliva, and how, in this manner, also, wholesome boils will be developed.

Generally, flow of saliva attends toothaches, and must, likewise, be maintained in the manner described, only that warm water must be taken in the mouth when the pains are violent, and meanwhile rub with cold water externally, and then lay the compress there again.

A radical cure from the susceptibility of toothache or from matters causing toothache, can only be effected by a radical water-cure, as also, generally speaking, it is not possible to cure an individual chronic complaint without at the same time stirring up all the other hidden morbific causes, and ridding the system of them. Thus it is that chronic cures are so tedious.

People who before have suffered of the toothache, get, in the water-cure, critical toothaches again, which differ from the usual ones in this respect, that they commence immediately with those symptoms with which the usual aches depart, namely, with secretion of an acrid, corrosive saliva, with swelling of the jaws or cheeks, and with the uncomfortable feeling, as if the teeth had become longer; then come gum-boils also, boils upon the external skin, and frequently such a soreness of the mouth that mastication becomes very painful. In such manner the organism rids itself, with the help of water, of the causes of past, and, also, of future possible pains, and the said critical symptoms are sufficient proofs that substantial foreign matters are the cause of all toothaches. After removal of these causes no cold can produce toothache, and this is also confirmed both by reason and experience. I am acquainted with several persons who formerly suffered terribly of this misery, but after having taken the water-cure have never again experienced the slightest inconvenience on that score, and laugh at the idea of taking cold.

Thus it is certain, that every one, who still possesses

good vital power, can, by the water-cure, rid himself for ever radically of this evil; just so certainly is it impossible to remove the pains *immediately*, because no true cure can be effected without pains. This last principle obtains not only in the physical, but also in the moral world.

The allopathic remedies for toothache consist chiefly in abstraction of blood and humor by leeches and drawing plaster. Concerning the first tappings, enough has already been said; those caused by the plaster are not less ineffectual and injurious. When corrosive and poisonous substances of a certain kind are applied in plasters to the skin, it absorbs from them, and, because they are poisons, it reacts against them by means of healthy juices; the juices are poisoned, and for that reason the organism expels them from itself. This executional procedure proves firstly, that in the "rational method of cure" anything is more easily found than rationality. Is there sense or reason therein, when it is the aim to cleanse the body of all impure matters, to force new impurities upon it, to compel it to turn its power of reaction away from the old against the new, or at least to divide it between both of them? When, therefore, a temporary mitigation ensues from these means, it is not because the original peccant matters have been thereby removed, but because the body has been deprived of the necessary energy. By reducing the strength of the body we can drive away all pains, and even life itself; and reduction of the strength is the universal remedy of allopathy for all acute pains and cramps.

Another kind of allopathic suppression of pain is to be reached by applying smarting substances to the hollow tooth, or to the gum. It is sufficiently well known, that these shameful remedies have not in all cases even a palliative effect, not to speak of their ever actually curing. Sometimes, for the first moment, the inward pain is deadened by the outward; but as soon as this painful reaction against the fresh poison is at an end, the strife with the old awakens again, which with the greater difficulty attains a result, the oftener it is disturbed.

When any person has been in the habit of using the above mentioned medicinal remedies for toothache, he has the best prospect of getting, sooner or later, a fistula in the gum, and accordingly the chance of losing a piece of his jaw-bone. When the endeavors to drive to the surface the matters causing toothache, by means of salivation and boils, are disturbed and suppressed by fresh poisons, the peccant matters at last gnaw internally, and generate internal festerings on the bones, which are called fistulas.

How can one best preserve his teeth, especially their whiteness and gloss? by what sort of powder? by which dentist?

This half toothless European race cannot any more without impertinence speak of their teeth, at the most of the ruins of their teeth, venerably moss-grown and crumbling ruins.

The teeth have three mortal enemies; first, everything that is poison, and medicine; second, everything that is hot; and third, all impurities of the stomach. The first two enemies corrode and break the enamel, and thus the teeth themselves; the third enemy covers the teeth with dirt and tartar, and this raises and presses them out of their sockets, so that they become loose and can fall out. Most powders are also injurious, which are used to cleanse and preserve the teeth, all so called tooth powders, because by their acidity they slowly destroy the enamel. Experience proves it; who has better teeth, the peasant girl, or the lady, that is, when you divest the latter of her ivory and porcelain? Instinct proves it equally as well, for these powders are unpleasant to the teeth, and sometimes even painful. Every substance, which occasions the body, or any part thereof, disagreeable or painful sensations, is unwholesome.

Whoever has cleansed his stomach by a course of water-treatment (en passant, I would advise every lady, whose mouth has not the fragrant odor of ambergris, to procure by help of water a rosy breath), and whoever adheres afterwards to a diet of cool foods (particularly smokes no tobacco), he will never resort again to the artificial means above spoken of; much rather he will live to see his teeth cleanse themselves entirely, and the tartar will be dissolved and passed off.

The only cleansing, which the teeth require, is done by the water, which occasionally passes about them in the course of drinking; whoever wishes to do it more radically may, after each meal, rinse and gargle his mouth with this delicious fluid.

Do you not believe it? Do you suppose the powders of the tooth breakers are sine qua non's? Then go hence and ask the tiger madam, what lotion she has to thank for her agreeably coquettish enamel; demand of the elephant what tooth doctor he employs, since a constant exchange is going on from his mouth into those of the beautiful ladies?

X.

GOUT.

As the rheumatism in its inflammatory form is with difficulty distinguished from real inflammation, so also in its chronic and atonic form the same difficulty in distinguishing it from the chronic and atonic gout. It is oftentimes difficult to determine, whether the face-ache is to be set down under fixed rheumatism or gout.

In these two diseases it is seen more clearly than anywhere else, that the classification of diseases in species and varieties is only an invention of the human mind, without possessing a corresponding reality in the external world.

Another question to be taken into consideration here is the hereditary nature of the gout, which is frequently asserted.

Besides the contagious chronic exanthematous diseases, there occur rarely, or not all, inherited perfect diseases, because by virtue of an admirably wise arrangement of nature, not the worst, but only the best juices of the mother, even when her body is deeply affected with disease, are conducted to the fœtus, and because the presence of material foreign causes is necessary to every complete and perfect disease.

But there are innate abnormities in the organism, and there are innate dispositions to diseases.

All substances impossible of assimilation (poisons), and all refuse portions of the body, are repelled by all the internal organs and parts, and in this manner are transmitted from hand to hand towards the skin and transpired; at least the organism endeavors to do this. But when by reason of insufficient activity of the skin it does not succeed in accomplishing this, these substances settle particularly in those organs, which are hereditarily the weakest, and in time bring on in that organ the disease which the father had, and which the son perhaps will have again.

The correctness of the view here presented is confirmed by the fact, that the "hereditary diseases" develope themselves usually in an advanced stage of life, oftentimes not till in advanced old age. Whoever follows the water diet, will certainly prevent any hereditary disease in himself, even if he has a decided predisposition thereto. Farthermore, it is evident, from this view of the subject, that "hereditary diseases" are curable by water, as this has also been already confirmed by experience.

We see certain families visited with lung complaints; all that is hereditary with them is weakness of the lungs; in consequence of which there arise at first in the lungs, from bad diet, obstructions (of refuse matters); in consequence of which acute efforts to rid themselves of these matters through cough or "inflammation;" in consequence of which medicine is administered; in consequence of which poison is deposited in the lungs, which sooner or later, as a last consequence, causes ulceration and death. It is precisely the same with hereditary gout. The gout is a disease of the bones and membranes which immediately surround the bones (periosteum). When these parts of the body are the weakest of all, the peccant matter deposits itself in them first of all, and generates the gout. The pains of the gout are produced by the foreign and poisonous matters exercising their destroying corrosive power on the membrane or skin of the bones. On account of this disturbance, the particles of the body intended to form new bony substance are in part not transformed in a normal manner into bone, and in part the waste matter of the bones is either not properly, or not at all, transmitted to the skin and transpired. Hence the cause of the gouty protuberances or knots explains itself, which are nothing else than the refuse of the affected bone.

The doctors have already made notice of this circumstance, that sometimes, when with gouty persons, after severe pains, a critical perspiration breaks out and becomes dry, the whole skin is visibly covered with white, earthy dust, as if with bone dust. Hence it follows without doubt, that material morbific causes, which the perspiration removes, are present in the gout. It is strange that the allopaths, who have in their books made mention of this circumstance, did not thence draw the very pertinent conclusion, that the gout could only be cured through activity of the skin, through sweating and boils.

At the present time the gout is called one of those diseases, which particularly is cured by the water treatment. It is universally a settled fact, that water cures with most certainty of the rude very material causes of disease, e. g. with much more certainty it cures of a mineral poisoning—mercury, steel, lead, copper—than a vegetable poisoning. The poison of belladonna is very particularly difficult to overcome.

The treatment of gout consists chiefly in sweat and douche-baths; that drives to the skin the accumulated morbid gouty matters, in critical sweatings, eruptions, and boils; still the cure is tedious, when the disease is old and deeply rooted. When it is happily ended, the recovered person, to remain healthy for the residue of his life, must adhere to the water diet; if he returns again to wine, coffee, &c., and particularly if he neglects a daily bath and washing, the old complaint will return again.

With gout the Allopaths even concede to the water-cure the possession of a certain curative power, and have already sent many of these patients to Graefenberg.

In the water-cure the critical sweats occur much more frequently and powerfully than in the old dry and medicinal régime, where such like critical perspirations appear but seldom, and only with strong constitutions. In the water-cure the critical perspiration covers the skin of the gout-patient sometimes for a length of time so considerably with a chalk-like substance, that any unaided eye may perceive it.

In gout the doctors assume a dyscrasy of the juices as cause of the disease, and derive this dyscrasy of the juices from false processes of preparation of blood and juice, so that consequently the digestive organs, by a false act of digestion, would make acrid and pain-generating humors from wholesome foods. Munde, in his so-called hydrotherapy, blindly follows this view. We can pardon the doctors for such an opinion, as they are placed by their instructors on a false basis directly in the commencement of their study; when one starts from false premises, he arrives necessarily at false conclusions. But when Mr. Munde, who, without having been filled and biassed with prejudices by a laborious course of study in a false science, had the opportunity of observing so many water-cures, still copies and repeats erroneous doctrines, whose falseness has been proved directly and practically by the results of the water-cure: he justifies his readers in the conclusion, that he lacks the mental ability, to deduct from the results of the water-cure the causal connexion of the processes of disease. In another place I will devote a few critical remarks to the last writings, and especially the hydrotherapie, of Dr. Munde.

The opinion, that the causes of diseases are of dynamic nature, and that the body can elaborate acrid matters and juices productive of severe pains from wholesome aliments, contradicts in the second place the laws of physiology, and in the third place the results of experience made by the water-cure.

(1) The position of philosophic view in regard to the doctrine of disease has already been given in the foregoing. If the causes of disease were immaterial and dynamic, they could not be recognised by any of the human senses, not even by any mental sense, and it would be an impossibility to avoid these causes. The human organism were then such an unfortunate abortive piece of workmanship, that it would not be a proof of the infinite wisdom, but of the surpassing stupidity of its creator; in the acceptation of the truth of the dynamic pathology, and of the medical therapie, the instinct of man were not only in vain, but would be a cause of his greatest unhappiness, and the production of unceasing confusion ; that same instinct, which dictates so unerringly to the most imperfect orders of creation the way to the maintenance of their life and health, which speaks just as loudly and distinctly in man as in beast ! Or has man perhaps less horror and disgust of poison than the beast has ? Has man less desire for food and drink than the beast ?

If, farther, the causes of diseases were dynamic, then every possibility of an investigation of the processes of disease as regards man is thereby rendered impossible, because as regards man the dynamic is inexplorable and incomprehensible. A pathology on dynamic basis is for the human mind a contradictio in adjecto, i. e. if it be required of such a pathology, that it shall contain truth. The homœopaths, who are much wiser, have comprehended all this very well, and accordingly never allow of any investigations and systematic expositions concerning the nature of diseases, and the causation of their processes.

(2) The physiological grounds against the acceptation, that the organism by an improper act of digestion can from wholesome foods and drinks generate such acridities, as brought by the circulation in contact with the nerves cause violent pains by reason of their corrosive power, are the following.

The transformation of the whole of a mild substance to an acrid and corrosive is not possible by any known chemical process; but substances, which are mixed with acridities, may be made corrosively acrid, by separating the mild qualifying parts, and thus leaving behind the corrosive. This last process indeed takes place during digestion, when foods and drinks are taken that are mixed with very sharp, pungent, or with poisonous substances. By the digestion, namely, the mild constituent parts are assimilated, the sharp pungent ingredients, on the contrary, pass separated from the milder unassimilated into the whole body at large, and produce pains by their contact with the nerves. It **is** precisely this process which produces by far the most cases of disease from taking poisons, with what constitutions we will see farther on. In this process, however, no acridities are *generated* by an improper digestion, but by an act of the most normal digestion they are ***separated*** from their mixture with mild substances.

Farther, combined poisons can, by chemical processes, be set free, or, more correctly speaking, there are mild substances, which, through chemical processes, can be transformed *partly* into corrosive and narcotic poisons; but the processes of digestion are so entirely different from them, that a change of mild substances into poisonous by false digestion must be called an impossibility, according to all known physiological and chemical laws. The most acrid substance, that the stomach can generate through disease from wholesome food, is the acid of the heartburn, but this is always very far from being a corrosive or narcotic substance; it does not contain, even in mixture, any of such like ingredients. Moreover, this acid manifests its presence to every one, who is affected with it, by its rising on the stomach. The great mass of gouty patients, however, are not affected with acidity of stomach, and the great mass of those thus affected, do not suffer of the gout. The acid of the stomach never contains by far such sharp substances as brandy, wine, and even beer; for all these drinks contain more or less alcoholic poisons; the stomach acid is, farthermore, by far not so sharp as the spices. It is therefore very strange to assume with persons, who eat all those sharp, pungent, and poison-containing substances, that the gouty and other pains are produced by contact of the nerves with acrimonious matters, which the stomach has made out of mild substances by false digestion. This assumption is still much more strange and irrational in the case of such persons as have taken, and still continue to take, unmixed poison under the name of medicine. Wherever poison is taken, there is sufficient material present for all conceivable sufferings and organic devastations, without being compelled to have recourse to, or being justified in the above considered hypothesis, which is wholly unfounded, and stands in contradiction with the known laws of physiology.

Farther on we will return to this subject again, that there is a disease of dyscrasy, or, more properly speaking, of false preparation of humors from wholesome foods; but we shall see, that also that disease is engendered through material causes, and that it does *not produce any corrosive and poisonous substances, but only faults in the chemical preparation of the blood,* consequently that its false preparation of humors is not of a positive but of a negative nature.

Here only the very sharp and corrosive substances come into consideration; for only by their contact with the nerves can internal pains of any kind be produced. Even the so-called nervous pains, the nervous toothache, headache, &c., are always of nervous-rheumatic or nervous-gouty disposition; the pain there is produced by contact of acrid substances with the nerves, and the nervous character of these pains arises from chronic disease and partial disorganization of the nerves. There are *convulsions, cramps, torments* of the nerves, which usually have arisen in some cases indirectly from poisoning, which, however, do not arise from direct and simultaneous contact with acrimonious foreign matters, when the secondary diseased state of the nerves is already perfectly formed. But every *actual pain* within the human body can be produced only by direct and simultaneous operation of foreign matters. These are mostly of a corrosive and poisonous nature; still there are pains within the body, that are not caused by chemical but by mechanical operation of the matters, for instance, the gravel pains by obstruction of various canals by means of stony concrements.

(3) The ground, which, from the results of the water-cure, opposes the assumption that the digestive organs of the gout-patient prepare the acrimonious pain-exciting humors, consists therein, that the said patients do not immediately in the beginning of the water-cure get critical vomiting or diarrhœa. When free* acrimonious matters are contained in the digestive canals, they are by copious use of water forthwith expelled through diarrhœa or vomiting, and vice versâ, where such evacuations do not ensue from the free use of water there are either no acridities at all, or, at least, no free acridities present. Such evacuations ensue immediately in the very commencement of the water-cure with those patients only who suffer of sour stomach, but by no means with the gout-patients. All what Mr. Munde says of temperance in his chapter on gout and otherwheres, borders much nearer upon the extreme of hunger, than the method of cure of V. Priessnitz on the extreme of over-eating. The truth does not lie half way between the two, but much nearer Priessnitz than Munde. I will not dispute that Priessnitz in most diseases allows his patients to eat too much and of too indigestible food; but Priessnitz deserves consideration on this account, because it is almost impossible for one who has never suffered from disease of the stomach or nerves, so to conform himself to these diseases that he can sympathize in all the different tones of these complaints. When Mr. Munde again warms up for our edifi-

* Free acrimonious matters mean here those old acridities that are not enveloped in slime, and adhere together with the slime to the walls of the digestive canals.

cation the story of Cornaro, and will show from his manner of life how little food a man requires, he overlooks the point that a man in Italy requires only half so much food as a man in Germany, and again in Italy much more than in India. According to my experience, only those patients in the water-cure when taking suitable exercise must not be allowed to satiate their appetites, who suffer of stomach or severe nervous complaints. My arthritical patients, who are not afflicted with either of these two complaints, I have always allowed, when taking proper exercise, to satisfy their appetite perfectly, and this is precisely the class of patients which I have as yet always radically cured.

The gout arises from sharp, pungent substances taken into the body from without; if these sharp substances be taken in any considerable quantity, *and if the bones and periostea especially in the joints are the weakest part of the body.* In that case the acrimonious matters and poisons of diet and medicine are more thrown off from the other organs, and, deposited on the bones and their investing membranes, impede the normal secretions and renovation of the bones, and cause thereby concrements of osseous matter. Still all this cannot occur until the organ of the skin becomes weakened, and this usually does not occur much before middle age.

It is my opinion, that with most gout-patients medicinal poisoning is indeed a co-operating cause of disease, but that a diet of sharp, high-seasoned foods, or of intoxicating drinks, is, however, the grand cause of gout, viz. under the pre-supposition, that the other internal organs are strong, and the bones, with their membranes, are hereditarily the weakest parts of the body.

The fully perfected gout returns mostly at fixed periods, generally in spring and autumn, when the body undertakes its chief renovation, and when therefore the deposited morbific matters are the most set free from their mucous envelopments, generate pains and disease, and cannot be excreted without pains.

The symptoms of the gout are well known in as far as they can be generally determined; they vary sometimes into the symptoms of other diseases, when the condition is a compound one. The symptoms of the pure and most usual gout are: a violent pain in the ligaments of the joints and the contiguous parts of the bones, accompanied by an inflammatory swelling and inflexibility of the joints.

The gout has different names, according to the different joints that are befallen therewith, as chiragra, podagra, gonagra (gout in the hands, feet, knees). Moreover, the gout has taken various denotations according to its various character; flying gout, settled gout, acute, chronic, atonic gout. Of these various characters of the gout, pretty much the same holds good as was said of the corresponding characters of the rheumatism.

The operation and effect of medical treatment of the gout are essentially as follows: The antiphlogistic remedies in arthritical fever produce the deleterious effects which are treated of under the chapter upon inflammatory fevers; the vomitives and purgatives ruin gradually the digestive canals; the narcotic poisons, as particularly opium (given to mitigate the pains), operate in the highest degree injuriously upon the nervous system, and fill the organism with powerful poisonous substances; the so-called antiarthritic medicines, as mercury, aconite, colchicum, camphor, cod-oil, &c., operate likewise decidedly prejudicially on the nerves and digestive organs, and impregnate the body with foreign matter; they do very great injury to the body, but the gout does very little; the gout triumphs over all these quackeries. Moreover, among the relatively enlightened portion of the doctors, the opinion prevails that the medical science is not capable of effecting anything against the gout.

The curability of the gout by the water-cure is already generally admitted, and therefore requires no farther demonstration.

I would classify gout into the true and false. The false gout, then, would be the pain in the bones, which is produced by powerful medicinal poisoning, particularly by a course of mercurial treatment; the true gout, on the contrary, would be the pain seated mostly in the articulations which is engendered by a faulty diet as the preponderating cause, when there is a predisposition to it that is a predominant weakness in the joints. According to my experience the true gout is cured in the water-cure chiefly through critical perspirations, the false on the other hand mostly through critical exanthems.

XI.

CHLOROSIS. SCROFULA. RACHITIS.

I HAVE already mentioned that there is in diseased digestive organs an act of false digestion, whereby the blood, and, indirectly, the other humors also are deteriorated. But, in the first place, the prime cause is always material disease-bringing substances, which are introduced from without into the body: with scrofulous, venereally diseased, consumptive, and arthritical mothers, this may occur to the fœtus even in their bodies; still, however, this comes into the world usually with predisposition only to scrofulous diseases, rarely or never with the disease perfectly formed. Secondly, such an elaboration of sickly fluids from the wholesome aliment never consists in this, that foreign substances of a corrosive or very acrid nature are engendered by a false act of digestion, but always herein, that either disproportions in the compounding of the chemical elements of the blood, &c., are present, or that one of these elements is entirely wanting. Thus, by this false act of digestion, no pain-producing substances are engendered.

The chlorosis, the scrofula, the rachitis, belong to the cachectic and dyscratic diseases; the mediciners also include pulmonary consumption, dropsy, venereal diseases, leprosy, and scurvy, erroneously under the same head.

(1) *Chlorosis.—Green Sickness.*—Symptoms of the disease are: pale skin, which sometimes darkens into a yellowish-green, and which is lax and of cool temperature; paleness and inflatedness of the lips; bluish rings about the eyes; depressed and irritable temperament; derangements in the digestion, and frequently palpitation of the heart with shortness of breath.

The nature of this disease consists in a diseased chemical constitution of the blood, connected with disease of the sexual organs, and frequently arising out of it.

The causes of this disease are usually several cooperating, as false diet, too much sitting, excessive exertion of the mind or of the imagination, medicinal disease, remains of disease from former scrofulous complaints, oftentimes also onanism.

The medical treatment consists mainly in the administration of bitter and aromatic remedies, rhubarb, muriate of ammonia, myrrh, but particularly iron and ferruginous mineral waters. The organism heals this disease sometimes despite medicinal treatment; frequently, however, such treatment causes it to run into hysteria, consumption, and dropsy.

The water-cure has already been proved in chlorosis; and, from many cases of experience, we can say that this disease is in every case radically cured by water, rightly applied, if no organic defects, particularly in the heart or abdomen, are present.

Chlorosis occurs only with the female sex, and usually in the years of sexual maturity.

(2) *Scrofula.*—The symptoms of this disease are a lax and transparent white skin, large and swollen abdomen, diseased and false appetite, feebleness and emaciation of the limbs, softness and flexibility of the bones, disproportionately large head, broad, almost square face, sunken eyes with dilated pupils and inclination to inflammation in them.

The hearth of this disease is to be found in the glands and the lymphatic system.

The medicinal treatment of scrofula operates, in general, much more injuriously upon the organism than medicaments employed in chlorosis. In scrofula more powerful poisons are given; as mercury, iodine, belladonna, hemlock; also, cod-oil, gold, lime-water, and the most various mineral and artificial baths. The organism can never attain to perfect cure under medical treatment; oftentimes scrofula is thus converted into tuberculous consumption, into hectic fever, consumption, and dropsy.

Under the water-cure scrofulous disease is *always* cured, whe1 it has not as yet been preceded by a medicinal course of treatment; aad even after this, it is cured by water when the medicinal disease has not laid too deep a hold upon the organs of life, and has not as yet exhausted the vital energy too much.

(3) *The Rachitis.*—This disease is nearly akin to scrofula, and likewise peculiar only to the age of childhood.

The symptoms of the disease are, large head, particularly the sutures of the head-bones being defectively united, enlarged abdomen, small limbs, swelling, and distortion of the bones.

Under medicinal treatment death most generally ensues through atrophy, or dropsy.

The correct hydriatic treatment cures the disease, when, as yet, no considerable medicinal disease is combined with it, and the organism not too much exhausted.

This frightful disease was, as very many others, quite unknown among mankind before the introduction of powerful poisons into medicine; consequently, not before the middle of the sixteenth century. In my opinion it can appear in no other children than those born of poisoned parents, especially of parents that have labored under venereal disease, itch, or scurvy medicinally treated.

XII.

HEMORRHOIDS, OR PILES.

The symptoms of this disease are, itching and burning in the anus, secretion of blood from the rectum, swellings and knots in the anus, discharges of slime from the rectum.

The piles accompanied by discharges of blood are

called bleeding, those discharging slime, the slimy—hemorrhoids; the knots, which discharge nothing, are called blind hemorrhoids.

The nature of this disease consists in a discharge of acrid matters, by transporting and eliminating them in blood; and, accordingly, the hemorrhoids, i. e. the bleeding, belong to the transition disease between the primary and secondary form. In the discharges, however, no general relief from old and new matters of disease is effected, but only partial from those acrimonious matters, which flow always anew into the body through drugging and false diet. The bleeding hemorrhoids are, by continuing in the use of medicine and false diet, converted, in the course of time, into blind, or slimy, or a metathesis of the disease occurs. Under the said deleterious influences the hemorrhoidal acrimonious humors are thrown upon the other parts of the body, and either find no discharge at all (latent hemorrhoids), or a discharge from the veins of the other organs, as, for instance, from the vagina and bladder.

Thus the effect of medicinal treatment upon this disease is a gradual conversion of the bleeding hemorrhoids into blind, slimy, and latent.

The effect of the water-cure is a change directly contrary, and, consequently, a cure of the bloody hemorrhoids by introducing no new acridities into the body, and removing the old in discharges of blood, critical transudations, abnormal secretions of urine, and exanthems. Of course, without corresponding diet no cure can be accomplished. Much exercise and adherence in the use of mild foods and drinks are the main requisitions of this diet.

The suppression of the bleeding hemorrhoids by medicinal remedies has always, sooner or later, the most disastrous consequences.

XIII.

SLEEPLESSNESS.

SLEEP is that condition of animals wherein the physical powers, together with the arbitrary voluntary motions, are in a state of perfect inactivity, and the susceptibility to perceptions of the senses is, to a certain degree, extinguished; wherein, on the other hand, the processes of circulation of the blood, of assimilation, of insensible perspiration, and of respiration, proceed regularly and undisturbed.

As the nature of vitality is unexplored, so also is the inward nature of sleep, of the suspension of several processes of vitality.

Sleeplessness, i. e. relative, can occur in healthy persons from want of exercise and satisfaction of the natural desires, which hinders the elaboration of the humors and the secretion of the surplus in seminal humors, and from these inducing in the organism a disturbance of its harmony, which is, in a certain sense, a state of disease.

Most conditions of disease disturb the sleep more or less, because in them abnormal processes are going on, which exceed the powers of the *sleeping* organism, or in other words, which are incompatible with the cessation of those functions, which are suspended during sleep. For this reason the processes of disease combat and resist sleep; when the former are in activity, the latter must yield, or be changed to a sort of half-slumbering; when the latter occurs, the former are compelled, for the time, to a full or relative cessation.

From the above it appears that sleeplessness is no proper kind of disease, *but that it may be an effect of all, and the most different processes of disease.*

Whoever suffers from sleeplessness without the above-mentioned cause of want of exercise, &c., in persons of full habit, and without painful or acute, or in general, marked symptoms of disease being perceptible, *with him there are, in the internal organism, latent organic deformations or ravages at work, and the sleeplessness proceeds from a reaction of the organism against the rapid extension of the disorganization.* The relative and imperfect reaction in secondary diseases is usually unaccompanied by symptoms, which come to the perception through the feeling of the patient, or are manifest to the physician; the absolute reaction in primary diseases is, on the contrary, always accompanied by such symptoms.

As fever is the effect of every exertion of the body which exceeds the conservative powers of the WAKING *organism, so sleeplessness is, in like manner, the effect of processes which exceed the powers of the* SLEEPING *organism.*

Hence, it follows that medicinal soporifics are, in a double sense, destructive in the highest degree; first, because they consist of stupefying poisons, and thus introduce poison into the body; and secondly, because they disturb the organism in its reaction against the rapid extension of an internal destruction or deformation already in progress.

Perhaps some one raises as an objection against the whole of my reasoning, that sleeplessness, at the present day, is a very wide-spread complaint, and that organic defects are not so widely extended.

To this I reply, that organic defects are just as widely extended as the secondary diseases are; in every chronically diseased person organic defects take place in the organs which are the seat of the chronic disease.

The dissections of corpses of those that have died of chronic disease, have also proved this equally as well as it has been proved already à priori, by true pathology.

It is in the highest degree ridiculous, when the doctors, by a post-mortem discovery of organic destructions and deformations, consider themselves justified in the event of the incurableness of the patient. *The presence of organic ravages in persons that have been medicinally treated in all the sicknesses which they have been subject to, is the most severe accusation imaginable against the medicinal method of cure.*

It is, in the highest degree, absurd to suppose the causes of organic ravages in man otherwise than in the poisons which they have taken. Wherever such poisons as the mediciners administer in the energetic diseases have been taken by the patients, there, evident causes are present for all conceivable organic ravages and deformations.

XV.

CHRONIC FEVER. CHRONIC NIGHT-SWEATS. DROPSY.

(1) *Chronic Fever.*—As the acute fever proceeds from the abnormal exertion which the organism makes to cast off accumulated matters of disease, an exertion which exceeds the normal powers, so the chronic slow fever pro-

ceeds therefrom, that the performance of the daily functions exceeds the strength of the machine, because one or more organs are being gradually destroyed by poison. Hence, we see that this fever is not the effect of a curative struggle, but of gradual subjugation, of the annihilation of the general system; hence, the fever is pitifully weak, as the thin pulse of such a patient evinces. With all yearlong medicine-eaters, the digestive organs are irritated and poisoned, and, consequently, such persons get a slight fever after every full meal, as proof that only by abnormal elevation of strength the operation of digestion can be accomplished.

(2) *Chronic Night-Sweats.*—The chronic night-sweats bear the same relation to the critical transudations as the chronic fever does to the acute fever. The critical perspirations in and after acute fevers, discharge the whole mass of accumulated matters of disease; on the contrary, the chronic eliminate nothing more than the daily refuse of the body, which naturally should be removed through insensible perspiration and respiration of the skin. Chronic perspirations are consequences of depressed deeply-ruined energy of skin, which is obliged to have recourse to the extraordinary assistance of sweating, to accomplish the business of excretion.

The issue of these diseased perspirations is oftentimes consumption, oftentimes dropsy.

In the case of chronic fevers, as well as of chronic perspiration, a slight chill follows every fever and perspiration; it rises to such a height at last that the body is constantly changing from one extreme to the other, because a relaxation must quite naturally ensue after the diseased over-strained exertion of the corporal powers.

The cure of these sad states of disease can only be effected by a tedious, troublesome course of water-cure; still, it is, in every case, attained with certainty when, as yet, youth, or sufficient vital energy is present.

(3) *Dropsy.*—This fearful disease claims more and more victims every year. What are its causes?

It can only be engendered through a double cause, viz. through poisoning and dry-skin régime (want of cold washing and bathing).

When the skin is so relaxed that it can no longer throw off the refuse humors which are daily deposited there from the internal parts, these fluids, which should have been transuded, accumulate under the skin, and produce bloatedness, paleness, and coldness,—the so-called dropsy of the skin.

The more a body is poisoned, the more need has it of abnormally free and copious transpiration, because it seeks thus to rid itself of its matters of disease and poison. Hence, it follows that in the case of poisoned subjects, a more than ordinary activity of skin is requisite, and that this important organ is, therefore, the first to become relaxed, if it is not sustained by the daily refreshment of cold water intended by nature. For this reason alone it follows that no one has more urgent need of cold-water-cure and water-diet than he who has taken much medicine. Hence, the well-known fact explains itself, that strong poisonings (be they either medicinal, and particularly those by mercury and china, or be they dietetic, from extravagant use of spirits, i. e. spirits of wine and alcohol in intoxicating drinks) very frequently cause death by dropsy.

When poisoning and relaxation of skin, and, consequently, disposition to dropsy, are present, contraction of a severe cold very often accelerates the outbreak of the disease, which otherwise might have lain dormant still a long time in the system; yet it is an error when some suppose that a cold might be the prime, or only, cause of dropsy.

When this disease is submitted to the operations of the hydriatic system in its commencement, it is always cured, if sufficient vital energy is still left in the body. The task of the cure is, so to animate the skin, re-invigorate it, that it again sets about its business of transudation. The critical removal of the already-accumulated fluids is generally effected by transudation or abnormal secretions of urine.

If the poisons that have been swallowed deposit themselves, particularly on an internal organ—perhaps because there was, during the acute disease in which the medicine was given, an elevated feverish excitement in that organ, and, consequently, determination of humors thither—then the last effect of the poisoning is either ulceration of this organ, or accumulation of stagnating fluid therein—local dropsy. The process by which this is effected is this: as protection against the penetrating poisonous matters, the organism sends, without intermission, its best humors and energies to the affected organ, partly to dilute the poisons, partly with and in these humors to transmit them to the skin and thence expel them from the body. In such manner their radical elimination can be gradually accomplished if water-diet, from within and without, be adhered in. If this, however, does not take place, and if the organ particularly burdened with poison loses its power to again throw off the humors pressing upon it, which become saturated with poisonous matter, so that they may be transmitted to the skin and removed by transpiration, then you have dropsy, whether it be on the brain, or the chest, or abdomen, &c.

Whoever casts aside medicine and intoxicating drinks and adheres to water-diet, is absolutely insured against the possibility of any kind of dropsy.

These local stagnations of serous fluid can be removed by the water-cure, when suitable vital energy still is present, and the disease has not, as yet, reached too high a degree of perfection.

The inadequateness of medicine to affect any of these diseases is well known, and the old curing art scarcely attempts to dissimulate here any longer; it confesses its weakness.

XVI.

CONCLUDING REMARKS UPON THE SECONDARY DISEASES.

When the medicinal poisons are taken into the stomach, they operate most injuriously upon the digestive organs, and engender secondary symptoms there in particular; when taken upon a full stomach, they pass, mixed with the food, into the chyme, into the chyle, into the blood, and through the circulation of the blood, into the whole organism, still unassimilated and remaining a foreign substance. By their admixture with chyle they operate less injuriously on the digestive organs; by this intermixture they are somewhat diluted and reduced, but more effectually conducted into the blood, than when they are taken into the empty stomach, in which a portion of the poison is retained and prevented passing into the blood by being enveloped in mucus.

The more powerful poisons are not given so frequently as the weaker, and the former cause pre-eminently organic destructions through ulcerations, through cancerous abscesses, and caries of the bones. The weaker poisons, which are administered in greater quantities, cause particularly dropsy. The poisons of common diet, especially the alcohol in intoxicating drinks, for this reason frequently produce dropsies of every kind, but never, of themselves alone, ulcerations of internal organs.

The medicaments of the class of corrosive poisons, as arsenic, mercury, concentrated acids, iodine, also, the many corrosive vegetables, cause particularly excessive stimulation, bluntness of the senses, deformation of the nerves, and dropsy.

The astringent poisons, as medicaments, cause particularly consumption, by obstruction of the finer canals, and by permanent contraction of the animal fibres.

The organic indurations, cartilaginous growths, ossifications, the disappearance and abnormal increase of individual organs, polypous growths, and strong concrements (in the gout and gravel-disease), all these painful and distressing organic defects and ravages, can be produced by poisoning only, which is, in most cases, the result of medicine, more seldom of diet, and most seldom the result of intentional poisoning.

All these organic deformations and ravages arise in the course of after-life, and generally, not before the years of middle or advanced age; the method of cure, under whose protection and influence such misery can arise, is already, for these reasons, in the eyes of every thinking man, marked and branded as a method of mischief of the most fearful kind.

All these disorganizations can be cured by water, and only in the first stadium, provided at the same time sufficient vital energy is present. Afterwards the water can only strengthen the organism and mitigate the organic disease. Therefore, let every one hasten to the water-cure as soon as he perceives the first symptoms of such disorganization. Every chronic affliction, and chronic sleeplessness, are symptoms of disorganizing processes within the body.

O.

THE CONTAGIOUS DISEASES.

THE epidemic diseases are oftentimes confounded with the contagious. The cholera, colic, yellow fever, are epidemic diseases; also, the intermitting and gastric fevers become so frequently.

All diseases that have a pure contagious character are, with the single exception of hydrophobia, attended with exanthems of the most various kinds.

In many of these exanthems, small worms or mites have been discovered through optical artificial assistance, which, in each different disease, have a different form.

It is highly probable, that these mites are not the effect of the exanthems, but the causes of them, and consequently also of the whole disease.

If any one introduces into his body any mineral, vegetable, or animal poison (with the exception of the poison of hydrophobia), it infuses itself into and extends itself throughout the whole circulation, and poisons thus the body; but in the same degree that the poison extends itself, and becomes diluted by admixture, in like ratio it loses its strength; it is also the same with the poison of serpents. In the contagious exanthematous diseases, however, the ratio is inverted; the smallest particle suffices to infect the whole organism, and then it generates the poison in much greater quantities than it has received it, *and this latter loses by its immense extension none of its strength.*

A production of acrid and corroding poison through physiological processes from the humors of the body is not only totally inexplicable, but it contradicts every philosophical conception of physiology and pathology.

But when we accept that the contagious exanthematous diseases are produced by animalcules, which are propagated according to the laws of animal procreation in the body of the infected person, then we arrive at not only an elucidation of that class of diseases now under consideration, but also preserve the philosophical basis in pathology and physiology. To this acceptation, therefore, we are mentally constrained, and that the more, since the perceptive power of the senses has already convinced itself of the existence of mites in the boils of the psora and venereal diseases.

Also, hydrophobia cannot be otherwise explained than by the hypothesis of animalic production of foreign being.

The contagious exanthematous diseases resolve themselves into two classes, into acute and chronic.

To the acute belong the measles, small-pox, &c. In these diseases we must suppose a species of animalculæ which, indeed, propagate themselves in the human body, but only for several generations, and which soon die off, where they do not quickly cause the death of the infected.

To the chronic contagious diseases belong the itch (psora), the scurvy, and the venereal diseases, &c. Here an animalcule (the magnifying glass has already detected it) must be assumed, which, under false diet and false method of cure, continues to propagate itself, till it causes the death of the infected by eating and gnawing continually deeper.

I must reserve for a later period entering into the detail of the contagious diseases, and here I must confine myself to what is said in the second edition of this work on venereal diseases.

In all diseases that are caused by inorganic matter, every medicinal poisoning can only result in injury without the possibility of any profit, without the possibility of destroying the matter of disease, because first, the medicament does not so penetrate the whole body as to reach all the secreted foreign atoms; and because, secondly, even if this were the case, still the solution of the inimical matter in nothing can never be effected. It is sufficiently well known that the annihilation of the smallest material atom is by no means possible, neither by fire nor by any chemical process. The apparent annihilation is nothing else than a reduction to its elements, or an entrance into other combinations. Hence, it follows with evident certainty, that the organism can never be freed of its causes of disease and foreign inimical substances otherwise than by their expulsion, that it is impossible to effect their annihilation in the body through medicinal means—it follows that every idea of cure by poison or medicine belongs to the most irrational and fearful of errors under which the human race has evei labored.

If, however, the causes of disease were really of immaterial and dynamic nature, as the mediciners of more recent date assume, then the idea of healing by poison, universally by the material, is still more absurd. In that case the cure would be possible only through dynamic influences and means, in some wise through Magnetism, Electricity, and such like.

Thus, in every case, whether corporeal matters or dynamic faults be the causes of disease, the medicinal science is as absurd and contradictory in its theory, as destroying and mischief-spreading in its practice.

It is otherwise with the chronic infectious exanthematous diseases, wherein the poisoning of the animalculæ of the boils, their acceleration from life to death, can most certainly be accomplished through poisoning the humors of the body. As soon as this has taken place the organism frees itself of the minute invisible corpses through transpiration and suppuration. This it endeavors to effect during the time of their life; but in this it could not succeed for two reasons; first, because they propagate themselves, and second, because they exert themselves unceasingly to work from the skin to the internal parts.

But the most fearful in this cure by medicine is, that the poison, which is given for that purpose, remains for the most part in the body of the poisoned person until his death, and gradually effects the annihilation, or, at least, the great injury of the internal organs, and thereby a distressing death by disease long before the natural age of man—unless this poison is eliminated by the water-cure. This elimination proceeds slowly, is attended with many pains, and, farthermore, few people are situated in circumstances which allow of a tedious treatment, dear in time and money. Hence this curing by medicine is one of the most direful calamities which can befall the human race.

In the acute exanthematous diseases—measles, small-pox, &c.—the medicinal poisoning is wholly useless (but not harmless), for this reason, that it cannot be discharged equally as soon as the disease decides itself; it requires many days before that poison, which is swallowed or rubbed into the skin, extends itself through the humors of the whole body.

The hydriatic treatment in infectious exanthematous diseases consists in sweat-baths, in compresses upon the parts touched by the exanthems, and in drinking.

Some have said, that the water-cure in itch and venereal diseases is exceedingly tedious; some authors have even asserted, that here water had proved itself insufficient, and that it is always necessary to have recourse to the specific medicaments. The first opinion is perfectly correct, if the infected persons have already been freely treated, or rather mistreated, with medicine before commencing the hydriatic treatment; for then cure does not depend alone upon destroying the infection, but also upon the elimination of the medicine administered, which must be retarded the more in proportion as the body through doctors' assistance has been robbed of its flesh and strength; the cure must also be retarded, if, besides the infection, there is present in the diseased body still an array of chronic affections, hemorrhoidal, arthritical, and others; for, as already said, the water cures no disease without at the same time setting in commotion all other hidden matters of disease.

The second opinion, in regard to the absolute insufficiency of water, can only be pronounced by such as are totally unacquainted with the hydriatic system, and whose stupid brain has as yet never been illumed by the faintest gleam of light on the nature of diseases and the operations of water upon the animal organism.

Numbers of persons, in the deepest miseries of secondary syphilis, have been radically cured at Graefenberg; among others, I am acquainted with a man, who, by the most horrible mistreatment of allopathic physicians, was plunged into the state of the last dreadful lues, who cast such an odor from his putrefying body, that the bath-attendants would serve him only in consideration of high extra-wages, who had scarcely a spot on his whole body on which there was not caries, or syphilitic sores, or mercurial disturbances, who, on his arrival, was carried from the wagon, for he could not stir a limb—and who still, under the hands of Priessnitz, acquired such health, and such a fulness of sound and solid flesh, as at the present day is seldom found among men. I would mention his name, were I not constrained to suppress it in consideration of the notorious character of the disease. He was a man known and respected by all his comrades, as one of the most substantial officers of the garrison of a large town; a solitary misstep had delivered him into the hands of his medical executioners, and they had so treated him, that they themselves, in the conviction of the absolute impossibility of his recovery, had sent him to Priessnitz. Several years after, when he was cured, meeting in a remote town with one of his executioners, who supposed him long since defunct and mouldered, and there presenting him reproachfully with his healthy figure, the doctor stared with horror upon this apparition, for he believed Beelzebub had sent thither the ghost of one of his murdered victims, and had with infernal irony given it the figure of a healthy man.

Yet, a word upon mercurial poisoning. Whether the mercury be swallowed or rubbed in the skin, it always penetrates into the substance and humors of the body. That it can never be assimilated to human flesh is tolerably well-known; consequently, it must either be driven off through the skin, little by little, or it remains as foreign gradually destroying essence—as poison. The allopaths presume to attract the mercury out of the body by warm sulphur-baths. It is seen, that allopathy is manifestly of the opinion, that a foreign matter is present in the organism; but the manner in which they will remove it, testifies to the grossest ignorance of nature's manner of cure. The sulphur, which has an affinity for mercury, will, they think, attract the mercury and neutralize it—as if the human body were a rag or sponge, without life of its own—as if the mercury so lay upon the surface, that it would be attracted by the sulphur. No, the affair is otherwise; when the sulphur presses in the skin, the organism must then defend itself against this new poison, and therefore has at that moment, least of all, the power to transmit to the skin the mercury hidden in the most internal and various parts of the body, and enveloped in mucus. The mercury remains rather where it is, and the sulphur, which penetrates into the body, must likewise be enveloped in mild mucus-like humors, because otherwise it would, like every other poison, destroy the nerves and all organs, into which it was transmitted. The whole consequence of the sulphur-baths, therefore, is this, that to the mercurial poison is superadded a new poisoning by sulphur. That this is so, has been incontestably proved by facts in the water-cure. All persons mercurially poisoned, who have subsequently passed through the sulphureous ordeal, have, in Graefenberg, always had the same course of crises; namely, their first critical transudations smell so decidedly sulphurous, that the bluntest olfactories cannot remain in doubt; when all the sulphur is removed, then follow perspirations of mercurial odors, also boils and eruptions and salivations, as surest proof of the secretion of mercury; frequently the syphilitic boils finally make their appearance again, which then, in a short time, are sweated and bathed away.

The warmth of these sulphur-baths contributes much to lower the condition of the mercurially-poisoned; for they render the body liable to take cold, which, in every poisoning, but especially in the mercurial, has consequences in the highest degree painful and fatally dangerous. All warm-baths, far from being able to effect a cure, rather weaken and effeminate the organism, and open the doors of disease. To health, and still more to cure, is necessary great activity and warmth of skin, a determination of humors externally, energetic life in the periphery of the body. By the warm-bath, however, the opposite of all this is gained; for, as the artificial action of it is to produce warmth of the skin, so, in consequence of the eternal laws of nature, the reaction after the bath produces coldness and relaxation of the skin. To this no contradiction is possible. Theory and experience prove it with equal force.

Still, although these truths are clear as the light of day, we see daily that many of the physicians prescribe warm-baths; is this to be imputed to their contractedness, or rather to a spirit of speculation, to insure work and pay for themselves in future?

P.

THE EXTERNAL, OR SURGICAL DISEASES.

UNDER this head I include only those injuries arising from external, mostly mechanical causes, but by no means those external exanthems arising from internal disease.

The external diseases, accordingly, consist in wounds, contusions, ruptures, fractures, dislocations, burnings, and freezings.

To heal such an injury the organism must deposit new flesh upon the injured spot, create new vessels to receive the minute new veins, &c.; in order to make this flesh it is necessary that it conducts thither to the injured part the material thereto—the creative humor, which is the blood—in abnormal quantity (in like manner plants heal an injury, a bruise, or cut), by transmitting the sap in great quantity to the affected spot; this abnormal flow of blood produces in the part to be healed an increased warmth, which can only rise to actual inflammation when the instinctive thirst of the wounded for cold water internally and externally is not appeased. Allopathy looks upon this determination of blood to the wounded spot, and the local vitality elevated even to a glowing heat, as disease, as a symptom that must be removed, and taps life's blood. Thereupon, the organism summons a fresh supply of blood thither, where it is needed, and the allopaths oftentimes continue their tapping, till the extremities are relieved of all their blood, and become cold; oftentimes, till the patient dies of debilitation (with internal inflammations also, they do the same), and then they have, in the most literal sense, slaughtered the patient.

When wounds, from the commencement, are treated with water, according to the method of Priessnitz, they heal readily, and always cleanly: these parts are never afterwards subject to pains, have no hard scar, or rather no perceptible scar, so that the spot where the wound has formerly been cannot be detected.

All wild animals operate similarly to Vincent Priessnitz; whence, forsooth, may dumb animals obtain such wisdom? All wild animals, when they are wounded, seek water; they soothe the heat internally and externally; and all wild animals heal their wounds much more skilfully than Diefenbach or Graefe: it is incredible, but every huntsman knows that it is true.

It would lead us here too far into detail if I should mention instances wherein among wild animals even some of those organic injuries, which we usually consider as decidedly fatal, are happily and radically cured. I have collected instances of the kind from the life of European park-hunters, and the trappers of the Far West, and intend to communicate these in another place.

It is highly probable that the beginnings of all medicinal art are to be sought in the application of herb poultices to external injuries.

As every organism endeavors to drive to the skin inimical matters that have penetrated internally, in like manner it endeavors, in a still higher degree, to cleanse wounds and sores of dirt and other matter by suppuration, before it closes and heals them.

The suppuration, as well with critical exanthems as with wounds and injuries, is nothing else than the assisting means whereby the matters of disease and of poison are carried off. It is impossible that the organism excrete these substances in their nakedness, minute and atom-like as they are, because, unenveloped in mild humors, they would affect the nerves painfully and dangerously in their passage towards the skin; indeed, without envelopment in a smooth and slippery substance, they could not be transported.* The critical transudation in the water-cure, always viscid, and of offensive odor, like suppuration from a sore, is, in its character, nothing more than a sort of suppuration, only that it is exuded little by little in innumerable little drops, from the millions of pores of the skin. When, on the contrary, the perspiration is not critical, i. e. does not contain any matters of disease, then it is fresh, not of offensive odor; also, it is rather watery than fat and glutinous.

In like manner as the internal curative struggles of the organism, the symptoms of acute disease can be suppressed by poisoning, thus can also the natural effort to cleanse a wound, by suppuration, and until this can be accomplished to keep it open, be overcome by external medicinal applications, and a closing and scarring of the wound be effected, contrary to the instinct and will of the

* Even when at table a crumb falls into the windpipe, mucus is instantly secreted, in order to make the crumb to be ejected, slippery and transportable.

organism. But it is ascertained to a certainty, that in all wounds artificially closed by salves, internal foreign matters become chronically fixed there.

The proof is this: all deeper and more considerable wounds and sores that are healed by medicinal art, leave, under the scar, a sensation of pain, or numbness and uncomfortableness, which is distinctly felt, either when the spot is subjected to slight pressure, or when a storm is approaching: with some it comes on, without any particular cause, at periodical intervals. Such artificially closed wounds oftentimes break open again in the water-cure, and then heal of themselves, disturbed by no salves and ointments, refreshed only with water. Then for ever afterwards every trace of pain or the least uncomfortableness has entirely disappeared. It has often happened that visibly material substances have been suppurated from such opened wounds; for instance, particles of meal, and even threads, and pieces of lint. Field wounds, that were of many years' standing, have again opened of themselves, at Graefenburg, and cast out the enemies and tormenting spirits.

As the medicinal art, so also the water-cure art, commenced by healing wounds; Priessnitz, the creator of the whole hydriatique, first cured particularly external injuries.

The treatment herein is various, according to the constitution and ailments of the patients; local baths, bandages, and drinking, accomplish the principal part. In the water-cure, it is impossible for a wound to close before it is perfectly clean and mature for healing. Particularly in thrust-wounds from three-edged weapons, the water is of invaluable worth, because in these wounds the premature superficial healing is of the worst consequences.

With animals, especially horses, water has been employed as a remedy in external injuries, for a long time, with the happiest consequences; one would be astonished at the results if, instead of the perverted manner formerly in vogue, the precepts of Priessnitz in this respect were to be followed. That would particularly benefit the poor horse; as man most prizes this noble beast, it is, next to himself, most honored with medicine; and the consequences of this poisoning are, in proportion, quite the same as with the human race. The delicateness and sickliness of the horse is universally known and regretted; people have so often lamented that the most beautiful of beasts should be the most sickly; it has never once occurred to the wisest of all animals that the sickliness and frailty of the noble race of horses is only an effect of medicine and effeminating treatment. Just in proportion as the races of horses are more or less poisoned by medicine, are they more diseased or more healthy. The English race-horse is almost as rheumatic and hysteric as a lady of rank; the peasant's horse is somewhat more rugged; still more so the polac, and the horse of the savage knows as little of disease as his rider.

When one understands how to employ water in wounds and injuries, then surgery is partially unnecessary, with the exception of setting dislocated joints, fractures, and other such seldom cases.

The surgical and operative help in cancers, growths and excrescences, caries, mortification, arterial tumors, and all other consequences of earlier medicinal poisoning, confines itself to the removal of the diseased part; the hydriatic assistance guarantees the cure and the preservation of the remaining part; this is the first small distinction between the efficaciousness of Priessnitz and of surgery; the second consists therein, that, after surgical aid alone, generally, the evil breaks out again in other places, while, on the contrary, the possibility and the root of every later mischief are totally extirpated by the water-cure. To be sure, in such cases, the water-treatment is very tedious, and a leg or a breast is cut away in a few minutes.

What a train of fearful errors: when an acute disease is fortunately cured into the body by medicine, the patient lauds the skilfulness of his doctor; yes, his heart is really touched with gratitude. When, after many years, the perpetrated poisoning developes its ravages and destructions, then it does not even occur to the unfortunate being that a long time ago his doctor sowed the poison-seed, which is now maturing to a harvest of internal ulcerations, of cancers, and unnatural growths. Now the sharp steel comes to the assistance to reap the fruit, to cut away the cancer; now the word is, go to some celebrated surgeon, and the refrain of all this wretchedness is the stupid exclamation,—how astonishingly advanced man is in science. "Life is short; art is long." Truly, indeed! and the longer art grows, the shorter grows life.

Q.

CRITICAL STATES IN THE WATER-CURE.

THE medicinal science understands by crisis, in the broader sense, the determination of the disease; by crisis, in the limited sense, the fortunate determination of the disease through evacuations, be they transudations, or mucous secretions, or exanthems, or depositions of abnormal matter in the urine, or diarrhœa, &c.

By lysis the said science understands so unimportant a crisis as escapes observation, perceptible only through its consequences.

From these explanations it will be perceived that the hydriatic has borrowed both the words from the medical science, and combines, with them, similar conceptions. It will farther be perceived that when, as is often the case, the mediciners deny to the lay of the profession the existence of crises, and accompany this denial with a compassionate smile, they make themselves guilty of a conscious falsehood. It is likewise falsehood when doctors misrepresent the acceptation of material causes of diseases as something in itself absurd, that, according to their assertion, only quite ignorant unprofessional men could stumble upon so unreasonable a supposition, because the so-called humoral pathology, which for a long time governed medicine, and which has still many adherents among the practical and older physicians, is based upon the acceptation of material causes of disease.

The hydriatique understands by crisis, the elimination of matters of disease in a manner perceptible to the senses, together with the excitation and fevers which often precede the elimination; it understands by lysis, the imperceptible excretion of these matters.

It has already been before shown how the water-cure system converts the chronic diseases into acute, viz. that the water, first of all, invigorates the organism, and then releases the enveloped morbific matters from the slime, and excretes them, oftentimes under raging fevers.

The conditions of disease during the water-cure, and particularly during the critical periods, are, throughout, different from everything which has formerly been witnessed. It cannot be otherwise, because this cure stirs up, little by little, all latent and most deeply-hidden matters of disease, and eliminates them through boils, &c.; on the contrary, all former methods of cure suppress the commotion of the struggles of disease, and force the causes of disease inwards. The essential distinction between water and medicine is, that the former drives the peccant matter out of the body; the latter, however, drives it into the body.

For this reason the mediciner seldom *perceives* that the causes of diseases are material; the water-doctor, however, makes this sensual perception in every disease. Hence arise the various views of the corporality and spirituality of the causes of disease. Whoever cannot, by any means, be convinced of the truth of the first view, for him it were advisable to go to Graefenberg ; there he *must* surrender, unless, in a genuine spiritual manner, he denies, to all perception of the senses, the power of furnishing proof.

To the characteristics of the critical conditions belong, first, the rare mixture of the joy of hope with pains of body, of which he alone has an idea who knows it through personal experience, although the solution of the apparent riddle is not difficult. The pain is produced by the aroused alarmed " matters," and the joy is caused by the instinct, which feels certain of cure, and is no more to be deluded and destroyed. One perceives in Graefenberg, in the fortunate one with whom the crisis has broken out, the lineaments of pain and of joy in picturesque contrast resting upon the same countenance ; one sees joy bursting from the eye, while the mouth laments and anathematizes the pains of the water-cure.

In many respects, one may speak of the pleasures of the Graefenberg state of sickness. What a pleasure to feel the appetite constantly growing, and soon to dare to eat whatever one wishes ! For it holds, as a fundamental position, that, after the instinct is again awakened, it is always the healthiest for every one to eat what he likes the most. What a freedom, farthermore, to dare to be always in the open air whenever one desires to be ; no possibility of taking cold ! What a delicious treat, always to dare to drink freely of the cool, limpid, mountain spring, when the fever-heat demands it ; to dare to plunge into a bath when the body, glowing like a Moloch, requires it, in order to bring into the world the crises, &c., which usher in the cure !

On the other hand, the treatment causes many troubles and pains; claims all the time set apart for pleasures; requires a more than usual perseverance. Of those who have fully accomplished the cure, many an one finds his expectations disappointed in a double respect. First, the cure (in many ailments) is more troublesome and painful than he had before thought possible; second, the results of the cure are, oftentimes, much more brilliant than the patient was before able to hope for.

Well observed, I speak of those that persevere until no crisis more will arise and can arise, because the body has been completely purified. Very many leave before this, and then do not carry out thoroughly enough the necessary after-cure. When any one has had a few crises with boils and discharge of suppuration, he is astonished already, that such a mass of bad humors was in his body, and thinks, surely, this must be the last. Still, it may be that, by farther use of the cure, the crises will be repeated again and again, until absolute purification and health are attained.

Much more disagreeable still than the boil crises is the cleansing-cure of badly slimed digestive canals; also, the matter here to be discharged is much greater in quantity. When a week has passed in vomiting and evacuation of slime, it appears a long time; where months thus pass away, the patient becomes desperate; still, he may live to see years pass away in this manner. This latter, indeed, is only a very extreme case, and then only possible when the coating of the bowels and stomach has begun almost with the first dawn of existence, and, therefore, it is so hardened that the gradual solution of it lays claim to so much time and energy of body. That the indurated slimings can be produced only by poison and medicine, and never by any other cause, on this subject there is nothing to be found in the instruction book of the rational art of poisoning.

In these stomach crises the patients sometimes taste decidedly the medicaments again which they have taken years before. In this, however, there is nothing strange; for the drug substances, which are preserved in indurated mucus, and to which neither water nor air can have access, retain their taste and peculiar smell as perfectly as if they lay in sealed vials. The same is the case with the poisons, which, divided into minute atoms, are chronically settled in the body; for instance, mercury retains its poisonous corrosive power when it has lain many years in the body, and then, by the water-cure, is thrown upon the skin; it eats both through the skin and the compresses also.

The first effects of the water-cure are, increased stimulation and an increased general feeling of well-being; so soon as the body has gained new strength, the crises commence, the burning fever, with the internal pains of the aroused matters of disease. In twelve to twenty-four hours after the commencement of this fever follows the outbreak of boils, eruptions, perspirations; that is—well observed, by proper continuation of the water-cure—always the course in chronic complaints. In common acute diseases the fever is relieved, much more promptly and surely, by the water-treatment, and the disease discharged in boils, &c., with still greater certainty, I say, because the acute disease is a curative effort of the body of its own accord, while, on the contrary, in chronic diseases, the organism must first be induced to the acute outbreak by a long course of water-treatment.

From that time onwards in which the Graefenberger water-cure begins to manifest its effects until the radical cure be accomplished, it is an occurrence observed by most patients, that the slightest injury of the skin causes suppuration, and is very slow of healing. This symptom is another proof to the point, that the water-cure draws the matters of disease from the internal to the external parts. One meets often in common life with persons of pale complexion, emaciated flesh, and other symptoms of chronic disease, whose skin however heals quickly, and without suppuration, after every injury. Hence, people conclude, that such a body must, by all means, possess healthy humors, and that such a person's miserable appearance arises from "weakness;" but that is far from the true mark; such a phenomenon proves that the evil lies in the internal organs and parts of the body. When such persons undertake the water-cure they learn the truth; in like ratio as their inward feelings improve, as their flesh hardens, the skin becomes more inclined to suppurations, until, at last, the genuine outbreak of the boils ensues.

All this is proof to this effect, that by the Graefenberg water-cure the vitality and energy of the exterior functions, and those lying nearer to the periphery of the body, are elevated in the same degree as the diseasedly increased activity of the internal noble organs is reduced to the normal condition; whence, then, the well-known fact explains itself, that the water-cure relieves, and finally, quite cures the passionateness of sick persons.

Gradually, as the cure elevates and invigorates the

organism, as the improved digestion supplies it with more blood, do the veins, the rivulets of the body, fill themselves, and their pulsation becomes full-toned; their flow, which before was crawling, becomes firm and sure. Every patient notices an entire change of pulse, if on entrance upon the cure it was not normal.

With many the change in the pulse sets in suddenly after a crisis. There is a sort of pulse-crisis, during which all the arteries beat and hammer, as if the body were a foundry. It circulates and chases through and around; it is a condition, as if the body were begetting a new body. This condition is promoted quite especially by much drinking. The reaction, after such a water-bout, produces more heat than an intoxication by wine; the body dilates, because all the veins course in the most swelling, fullest tempo, and because the water presses mechanically from the interior towards the exterior. The skin is very hot, and that is always an agreeable feeling—(only the internal heat is oppressive)—one feels in the skin a prickling and stitching, which arises from the transudation of acrid matters of disease. This is always the best feature with such a water-debauch, that no nauseousness, or other disagreeable consequence, follows in its course, but rather it arouses keen hunger, and a high tone of stomach. Drinking is a chief requisition of the cure; still, there is here also a too-much, if one continually pours down water against the indications of instinct.

As the pulsation of the blood, so also the color of the same is altered by the water; from the melancholy deep-red, it passes to the bright light shade which we see gush from the veins of the stricken deer. Water makes ruddy blood, and this transparent color is, together with the increase of the blood and the purification of the skin, the cause of the rosy color which the complexion gains by the water-cure.

R.

WHAT DISEASES ARE CURABLE BY WATER?

ANSWER :—All kinds of diseases are curable, but not all degrees of disease, and consequently not all sick persons. Whoever is curable to-day, he is next year, or, perhaps, even to-morrow, no more so.

All kinds of disease are, for this reason, curable, because they are engendered by material causes, *and because the organism, and all and each of its organs, possess the power of excreting all kinds of foreign matter.*

Accordingly, not water, but the organic strength, is the universal remedy for all diseases, which strength can only develope itself victoriously when all the requisitions of the organic instinct are satisfied, and the objects of its antipathies withdrawn and withheld.

But all *degrees* of disease are, for this reason, not curable, because only that state of disease is curable *in which the organic power is stronger than the power of the matters of disease.*

Accordingly, the hydropath, who is to determine upon the curableness of the patient, must more necessarily be acquainted with the degree of the disease and the measure of the organic strength, than with the variety or character of the disease.

S.

AN INVITATION TO THE PHYSICIANS.

I CHALLENGE all the physicians of Germany, and, if needs be, of all Europe, to disprove my doctrine of disease. If any one convinces me that the doctrines of this book are erroneous, like all those heretofore published, I will confess the same honestly and publicly ; if any one produces ingenious sophisms, or plausible arguments, against me, I will disprove them ; if any one comes out against me with uncommonly abusive language and unfair polemic, I will not notice him.

Only one request I would prefer : if you accept my offer, I beg you, leave the learned jargon of your craft at home ! Believe me, the times are past in which the public doffed their hats to your kitchen-Greek words of classification, in which it let itself be imposed upon by the charlatan jingling of senseless hollow expressions after the manner of metaphysics. Every truth that profits mankind, every truth, that evidently is truth, must so be brought forward, that every unprejudiced human understanding, every thinking human head may comprehend and hold fast to it.

Truth is like the pure mountain water in transparency, and refreshing invigoration; in its first effect it is like to the lightning's flash, which fires and illuminates; in its after effect, it is like to the whole storm, which purifies the atmosphere, and revives every living thing.

When any one brings forward a doctrine or a book, containing hard-digestible matters, it is half or whole errors, indigestible as well by the author as by the reader. That is, in every case, an unprofitable book, which a thinking man must twice read in order to understand. Not only must the reader comprehend the book, but the book must also be inviting to the reader.

But when it comes to writing upon subjects of which the writer himself has no conception, which, perhaps, are beyond the conception of mankind; then, one requires of necessity a deep, learned style and metaphysical phraseology, in order that absurdity may appear like sound sense.

THE END.

APPENDIX.

DIETETICS AND SEA BATHING.

THE human race of the present day is striving after mental rejuvenescence. They should first become corporeally young and healthy, and cast off their flannel doublets and woollen jackets; and, especially, beget for themselves a new skin in the cold bath.

Hitherto, I have only spoken as to the manner in which people are to cure themselves of diseases, and will now declare my opinion of the manner in which people may protect themselves against the diseases of the future.

In the morning when you awake, spring hastily out of bed, as if you were already booted and spurred for the chase, and refresh your skin with a cold bath. Whoever cannot do this, let him have a pail of water dashed over his body, or wash the entire body with a wet sponge or towel—that every one can do.

If you are not thoroughly warm when you awake, upon getting out of bed rub the skin of your body with your hands, until it is very warm, and then bathe.

After the bath, take exercise in the open air, until the reaction of warmth has completely returned: if this feeling of comfortableness passes off after you have returned home from exercise, cover yourself up warmly with comfortables, until the most perfect reaction has been produced.

After the walk, or exercise, breakfast from bread and butter and unboiled cold milk, unskimmed and as fresh as possible.

Here a remark as to the coldness of foods and drinks.

All warm food and drink debilitates the stomach, but cold invigorates it. To be sure, the first period of the transition from warm diet to cold is extremely sensitive and disagreeable to the stomach; but soon it becomes a habit, and promotes the vigor of the digestive organs in a wonderful manner. The reason why the cold strengthens the stomach, is the same as with the skin. When any thing warm comes in contact with the skin, or is taken into the stomach, the first effect is an elevated temperature; on this account the reaction, which always strives to produce a contrary effect, causes in this case a depressed temperature and depressed energy. With cold, however, the converse is the case; in addition to this highly beneficial reaction of warmth, and consequently elevated energy, the cold performs also the office of constringing the fibres of the stomach and skin.

The experience of Graefenberg has most perfectly established the beneficial effect of cold, or, at least, quite cool food; individuals who suffered of very great weakness of the digestive organs, were restored by a continued course of cold diet.

Now for the defence of milk.

The general opinion is that milk slimes or engenders mucus in the stomach: that objection, however, can only be raised against boiled milk. As soon as one has accustomed himself to unboiled milk, he is sensible of its beneficial effect upon the stomach; moreover, it contains the most wholesome of all alimentary substances, and exerts an excellent effect as an antidote against acrid humors, as also against inveterate and recent medicinal poisoning.

Whoever cannot overcome a dislike to unboiled milk, should breakfast either from bread and butter and water only, and replace the milk by cold roast meat, or whatever else is agreeable to his taste, provided it is nothing that has undergone fermentation, or nothing imported from a foreign zone—particularly no coffee.

For this reason, I am opposed to all outlandish articles of food:

The edible products of a zone are wholesome only in their native zone

I needed the observations of long and distant travels to perceive these maxims of nature. Priessnitz, with his medicinal instinct, appreciated it without quitting the horizon of his own blue mountains.

In the far North, fat grows in abundance, but no hot and stimulating vegetables. Therefore, when you are in Lapland, eat a sufficiency of fat to protect yourself against the effects of cold; but eschew eating all spices—they destroy by inflammation.

In the hot regions of the South, fat is wanting to the animal kingdom; the vegetable kingdom produces hot spices. Therefore, if you do not eat lean food and spice upon the Moluccas, you become the certain sacrifice to a disease whose seat is in the stomach and bowels.

It is impossible for any one to dispute these doctrines of experience; neither can any one take exception to the conclusion which I have thence deduced; and thus it must be admitted, that people should avoid the products of foreign zones, if they would eat and drink what is wholesome.

Therefore, resign your coffee and resign your tea, until you go to Arabia and China; there you may sip thereof to your heart's desire—there it will agree with you.

The injuriousness of fermented and intoxicating drinks is disputed by no one. Still, people frequently say, "taken in moderation they do no injury." That is, however, a deception: taken in moderation they do moderate injury. Therefore, let not wine become a daily necessity; and if you drink it on rare occasions, drink at the same time much water.

If the intoxicating drinks were not of themselves injurious, still their daily use would be dangerous, on account of their frequent adulteration and occasional poisoning.

Thus far I harmonize with Priessnitz—now comes the divergence. At dinner I would not willingly dine with him off of his dishes. At dinner, Priessnitz is a true German of the old school; he recommends household fare, however, with exclusion of all smoked and salted meat, all salt preserves, such as herrings, sardelles, etc.

Salt meat must be avoided for more than one reason. This kind of food introduces so many acridities into the body, that a healthy person has enough to do to get rid of them—even if he should be so fortunate; much less can a body that has long been afflicted with matters of disease or diseased humors, even think, while under the salt diet, of overcoming and improving them. Still more, the salted articles are injurious to the stomach, and stand in like category with the bitter stomachics, of which further on. Thirdly, salt meat contains but a very small amount of nourishment, as every chemist can prove to an evident certainty. The nutritious quality of meat consists in the juice or gluten, not in the fibre; this juice, however, the brine extracts and absorbs. Still, the public in general are of the contrary opinion. They consider this meat to be very nourishing, for this reason—because it remains a long time in the stomach; without considering that this quality is owing merely to its indigestibility. Finally, this food is of an unsweet odor, offensive to a delicate sense of smell, disgusting to a refined palate.

Leave salt meat to the sailor. He has nothing else, and he can best make away with it, because his whole general mode of life—the sea air, the daily involuntary bath, the exercise—metamorphoses him into a sort of shark.

Priessnitz gives his patients—even the dyspeptic—besides baked meat, also boiled meat. He appears—like all the inhabitants of Southern Germany, and also the majority of those of Northern Germany—to have no idea of the preparation of roast meat. That they learn only from the English, which always finds a place upon their well-supplied tables.

"When a soup has been boiled out of a piece of meat, it is then suitable for dogs, but not for the human stomach." Thus the English judge, and rightly; for such meat contains but little nourishment, difficult of digestion, and so disrelishing to a civilized palate, that dry bread is far preferable to it.

The meat should be roasted, and in such a manner that it may still retain internally the red color of the juice of the meat. Thus only is it sweet and relishing, easily digestible, easily masticated, and very nutritious. But if people roast their meat, after the manner of their grandfathers, for hours together, the ruddy juice evaporates, and is consumed by the atmosphere in the form of gas.

Still, it is requisite that meat, for a good roasting piece, be taken from a young animal. But if this is not to be had, how then? Then eat, much rather, only vegetables and farinaceous dishes, etc.

The roast beef of an Austrian kitchen is precisely the opposite of what I have represented as the *ideal* of a roast.

In Germany, in badly-managed households, people go so far as to first extract a soup from the predestined roasting piece. Such a procedure is not merely reprehensible, it is criminal treatment of any refined guest, an insult.

Priessnitz excludes no kind of animal from his diet table; he allows, also, the hard-digestible pork, duck, and goose. To eat of these unclean animals is ungenteel; however, of that we are not speaking here; I believe their flesh is not wholesome. If it does not produce any distinct disease, still it vitiates the humors of the body. Great Moses! great Rumohr! why have you not the power to give laws to the German kitchen? Herr von Rumohr says, in his "Spirit of the Culinary Art," although one may not ask quite too much of a gentleman, still he may require that he eat no hog's flesh.

Also, Priessnitz does not recommend the flesh of wild animals, as venison, etc., because it creates too much blood. It is inexplicable to me, how a man of such natural acuteness should give the preference to domestic animals over the wild, free-roving denizens of the forest—to these tame animals, that are fatted among the dung, and fettered to the stalls of a barn, deprived of all exercise, and sometimes also of pure air! And how, then? Is blood a disease? Too much blood? And that in a water-regimen? No! long live venison and game; or, rather, let them be destroyed, so that we may eat them!

At the vegetable dish Priessnitz is again a German, down to the very sour-krout. Whoever has been so unfortunate as myself, to have been sick and compelled to go to Graefenberg, he may there experience the following meal: 1. Baked beef, which is always first parboiled to furnish a soup, and onion sauce! 2. Roast pork and sour-krout! 3. Tyrolean apple-strudel (a sort of colossal apple dumpling, made of dough a little shortened, and fried in a sea of fat), and curd cake!—and (mankind can endure a great deal) live through it, since he has no choice.

Priessnitz warns all those of weak stomach against soup; people should go further, and banish all soup entirely from the table. Soup makes too slight an impression upon the relaxed walls of the stomach, to arouse their energy. But *warm* soup, in particular, weakens the stomach. All soup is, for this second reason, not healthy, because it occupies the space which should be occupied by water. Cold water is the most important of all promoters of digestion, for the simple reason, that it best aids the stomach in macerating its foods, in extracting from them their nutritious properties, and because, secondly, by means of the reaction so often spoken of, it produces the requisite and *permanent* elevated warmth of the stomach.

On the contrary, soup does not decompound the foods in the stomach: soup must be decomposed itself, and that is too great a demand upon the gastric juice.

"But how? Have indeed broths been for centuries past recommended to sick people, and is that suddenly to be pronounced wrong which has obtained as truth since the times of our grandfathers?"

I pray you, good aunty, spare me such objections. For centuries the practice of burning witches was in vogue, and yet a witch never existed.

Oh, that people would only pay some regard to their human instinct! All patients in acute disease thirst after cold water to drink! All weakness of stomach manifests a repugnance to soup!

Instead of such a dinner, I propose the following:

First—No soup, and but *one principal* dish; because the stomach digests a similiar quantity with greater facility, when it consists of a simple quality, than of a compound; and because, in cases of weak stomach, the temptation to eat too much is greatly increased by a multiplicity of dishes.

Second—Let this *one* dish consist of a piece of well roasted meat from a respectable animal, most preferably of venison or game, then of young beef or fowls, then mutton, veal, etc. This roast meat to be accompanied either by stewed green or dry fruit, or a vegetable, as rice, potatoes, salad, or any thing else that has not an unsavory odor, such as cabbage. The principle is well established, *that whatever smells bad, is difficult of digestion, and not wholesome.* Do you believe, then, Nature has given to man his noble nose to no purpose?

Third—After the roast, nothing but good bread and butter, and sweet, unboiled milk, or, in summer, rich, curdled, unskimmed milk, or raw fruit.

Females generally prefer farinaceous preparations, and these are as serviceable to them as meat to man. Then, the whole meal of a female may consist of farinaceous preparations, with fruit, and bread and milk.

At Graefenberg, the evening meal consists of bread and butter and milk only, which, however, is devoured in extensive quantities. When people sup two to three hours, they may also take a little cold beef, or fish, or farinaceous pudding.

When I also say, drink nothing but water and milk, accustom yourselves to drink considerable water, take much exercise, sit little, rather stand or recline—then I have concluded the rules for the day's work.

Now, ye gourmands, who are given to wine and chocolate, to spices and Parmesan cheese, to caviar and to the sardelle, can you dispute the wholesomeness of this natural diet?

Or do ye smile as epicures, and thank me for my advice, because it robs you of all pleasures of the palate?

Believe it not! Else I must serve you with an answer which would shame your understanding!

Only do not suppose that ye are epicureans. Epicurus was a very sensible man, and would have been ashamed of such disciples.

Epicurism is wisdom; but your epicurism is a very contracted epicurism! It is an epicurism which one can at the most excuse in the understanding of a child.

Whoever wishes to carry the enjoyment of every perception and pleasure to the greatest height, let him be aware of the fact, and never forget it, *that the magnitude of the enjoyment depends upon the susceptibility for the perception of the enjoyment, and not upon the object of enjoyment.*

The diet which I have described, sharpens the senses in an astonishing degree; it steels and strengthens the body; but in order to be able to enjoy things truly, delicately, and extensively, and constantly, one requires extremely delicate senses and robust health, and strength of body.

This diet sharpens particularly the senses of smell and taste to such a delicateness, that the instinct, long destroyed by the usual diet, awakes again in the man, and serves its master as an infallible private physician. Whoever, in delicateness of the palate, has become possessed of true instinct, he may, in sickness and health, always follow the propensities of his appetite.

That part of the instinct which serves to the *maintenance* of the animal life, resides in the senses of smell and taste; this instinct nature has bestowed upon both man and beast in like degree of keenness and infallibility. The nose of a natural man points out to him every poisonous plant, still more so the sense of taste. To destroy this instinct of the nose, the use of warm food and drink is alone sufficient, but the use of the stupefying weed, tobacco, is more than sufficient. In like manner, the scent of the hound becomes obtuse from eating warm food, as every huntsman knows.

I am well aware of the dogma, which originated in the myoptic wisdom of the old-fashioned spectacled magi—"Instinct was given to the beast, but understanding to man."

The beast also has understanding, has the power of comprehending and obey ing: aye, the nobler animals possess even the noble faculty of fancy.

Does some one ask, If the most simple diet warrants the greatest number of enjoyments, how were it possible that man could stray from the diet of nature to the diet of refinery?

That were possible for this reason: *because the brief transition from the natural to the unnatural supplies more enjoyment than nature vouchsafes.* That is a great truth, which ought to be published in giant letters.

Since the increased quantum of enjoyment continues only during the progression of the transition, it sinks the transgressor deeper and deeper, until his senses and the capability of enjoyment are rendered so obtuse, that he happily arrives at Cayenne pepper and aqua-fortis.

With virtue and vice it is quite the same. As the transition from the natural to the unnatural creates the highest intoxication of enjoyment, so the return from the unnatural to the natural gives rise to the most bitter sufferings and deprivations; consequently, a heroism of purpose is necessary to this conversion. But soon, very soon, the conflict has been maintained, and, as recompense therefor, happiness is again restored.

In Graefenberg, inveterate gourmands of the finest, or rather of the coarsest kind, have been brought to the confession, that never before had their port wine and sardelles at breakfast tasted so delicious to them, as now simple milk and bread. The resurrection of the delicateness of the palate ensues at a much earlier period than one would suppose.

What can you reply, you refiners, who arrogate the name of epicureans?

The delicate palate perceives in milk the stimulant and the spice which your coarser palate seeks in Cogniac and Jamaica; the delicate palate can speak of the aroma and flower of milk.

Do you presume upon possessing a nicety of taste? Nicety of taste! You! Your coarse, obtuse palates can be deceived by disgusting, spoiled food, if you only do not spare the biting buck, which you call sauces. That occurs daily without your being inwardly aware of it.

CLOTHING.

Do not wear woollen garments next to the bare skin; wool excites the skin to perspiration, and one should avoid perspiration, except when one intends bathing after it.

In Graefenberg, even feeble and aged persons have always, within two weeks, in inclement seasons, laid aside their woollen jackets, which were so old, that they might well celebrate their jubilee.

Accustom yourself to light clothing, but do no violence to yourself. If you are in general inclined to feel cold, if you have no comfortable warmth of the skin, that is a proof that you harbor matters of disease in your internal organs. and that the central functions have gained a preponderating energy over the peripheric. You need a systematic water-treatment; you will be cured by boils.

PASSIONS.

During the actual cure avoid every excitement. Priessnitz, therefore, strictly prohibits all playing for money, all unreasonable desires of the fancy, still more the actual enjoyment of sensual love; he admonishes against anger, vexation, envy, etc. Also, such patients as have only local affections, and otherwise blooming health, he sentences to celibacy, as long as the actual treatment continues.

DIET FOR DISORDERED AND DYSPEPTIC STOMACHS.

In Germany, people are not exactly very moderate and healthy eaters, neither are they very moderate drinkers, only they drink no water. Consequently, stomach disorderments are a part of the daily business of a genuine German, and belong to the chapter on diet.

The remedy par excellence for invigoration and purification of the stomach, is cold water; for this purpose, if it is to dissolve old slime and produce vomiting or purging, it must be drunk constantly in large quantities.

The allopathic tonics, bitters, and piquants, are the sworn mortal enemies of the stomach.

This error of the doctors has arisen thus: those bitters and piquants, as indigestibilities, excite an elevated activity in the stomach, in a certain measure an acute struggle of disease, in order to overpower and eject the mortal enemy. On the occasion of this struggle, the stomach powerfully digests its contents, or, when it is empty, it manifests an earnest desire after food, as a relief, and, to a certain degree, as a fortification against the enemy. One perceives this is no digestion and no appetite of health, but of compulsion and necessity.

Does some one say, every energy must have an enemy, in order not to become torpid; and for this reason bitter things are wholesome? I reply, firstly, the enemy must be such an one, that he can be overcome; but that is, in this case, not possible, because those bitter things are absolutely indigestible; a superior enemy discomfits his antagonist. Secondly, with the stomach it is really unnecessary to create work for it artificially—it has already enough naturally.

When this same procedure of stomach-invigoration is daily repeated, the stomach sinks daily more and more deeply into the irrecoverable misery. Then another danger also arises. In order to carry off indigestibilities, also to protect itself against the pain which they occasion, the stomach has recourse to slime, or mucus, wherein it envelopes them. If it is compelled to do this daily, its power becomes crippled; it prepares the slime, but cannot again purify itself of it; the stomach gets coated with slime, and mucous growths arise. Now the patient experiences an incessant oppression in the stomach, and periodical nausea. The doctor administers purgatives and vomitives; the latter have no result, and the former cause nothing but discharges of mucus, which each purgation causes to be newly prepared for the purpose of carrying off the poison of the purgative. Hence, the doctor concludes the stomach is clean, but only weak, and must be strengthened. Piquant, and sharp and biting substances exercise a similar evil effect upon the stomach, from similar grounds; they excite an elevated energy, because they torture the stomach; they themselves, however, are indigestible.

Even table salt, used in excessive quantities, belongs in this same category. People must salt their foods only moderately, if they would not produce acridity of the humors of the body, and weakness of stomach.

Whoever has taken much of allopathics, tonics, or other stomach-destroying medicaments, may, if he has the symptoms of oppression at the stomach, and of repeated nausea, be assured that his trouble consists not alone in weakness of stomach, but in a coating of the stomach with the toughest slime ;* neither should he let himself be deceived by the unsuccessfulness of purgatives ; the powerlessness of these and other medical remedies has been already spoken of.

When patients of this kind are not yet too old and weak, they are, by perseverance, surely cured by water, and they will be themselves astonished at the quantities of slime which they throw off.

For this purpose, water must be drunk in considerable quantity ; the stomach soon accustoms itself to it. It is, however, necessary, together with much water-drinking, to take a daily cold bath, so that the central functions may attain a ruinous preponderance over the peripheric ; still more, daily clysters and sitz-baths are necessary.

Such a treatment for inveterate slimings is very tedious ; months may elapse before the first trace of solution of slime ensues, and the period of purification with vomiting and purging may continue months longer. Whoever endeavors to abridge this period by means of medicinal purgatives, destroys the cure, and brings himself again into the old misery.

In order to learn what is necessary for a sick stomach, one should not go to extraordinarily learned professors, but to quite unlearned dogs, devoid of all titles. The dog, when his stomach is deranged, drinks water until he vomits or purges, and then he feels well again.

Here I would take the opportunity of warning all against an error which is, in the highest degree, injurious in its consequences. Some persons presume to assist a weak stomach by sparing it from labor, inasmuch as they feed it upon pure nourishment contained in the strongest broths, raw yolks of eggs, etc. That is the surest road to complete ruin. When one endeavors to spare an organ the activity which nature has designed for it, it soon goes to its final rest.

---

* These symptoms are, without doubt, unerring indications of mucous or slimy coating of the stomach ; but their absence is no guaranty of a pure stomach. Very inveterate mucous coatings may exist without those symptoms, and always do exist, if the symptoms have existed in earlier years. After a mass of slime has been fixed in one spot for several days, without the assistance of water it remains there, in every case, until death. Still, it grows so hard that the nauseousness may quite disappear ; and when it is not extensive, its effects upon the health are imperceptible. Even when it is so extensive as to cause life-long paleness and considerable emaciation, yet, for years, every trace of a diseased feeling in the stomach may be wanting. However, at last it produces death, by marasmus, consumption, or ossification of the digestive canals, or miserere.

BATHS.

Before I ever heard of Priessnitz or Oertel, I knew that daily cold baths were necessary to health. The woods, and the wild animal nature therein, had taught me that. That is, I reflected how it was that cultivated life was so entirely different from the natural life. I reflected how it were possible to replace by art the healthfulness of the natural mode of life. Every creature is bathed daily in the dew, or rain, or snow, or in the river, or sea; consequently I concluded the cold bath must be very healthy.

Further—in natural life the most cold water comes in contact with the feet and inferior parts of the body; consequently, it must be necessary to wet the feet and legs more with water than the body. Also, this last conclusion I find beautifully justified by the theory which I have learned at Graefenberg. For it is a principle in my theory, that wherever the water is most abundantly and frequently applied, thither particularly it conducts energy, warmth, the matters of disease, and the discharge by boils. "Feet warm, head cool," that we have long understood; but not how to attain it. Thus, then, by bathing the head least, but the feet most of all parts of the body.

This principle explains how it is that, with most men, all acrid matters deposit themselves in pimples upon the skin of the face. Because most men are so uncleanly as to wash daily nothing but the face, and not the whole body. Females should, if only from considerations of beauty, take daily a cold bath, and also another foot bath; then the pimples and freckles would certainly throw themselves upon the feet and legs.

The most excellent of all cosmetics is common spring water. It imparts fresh ruddiness, cleanliness, and a kind of transparency to the skin. It gives to the evaporations of the skin a peculiarly sweet and delicate odor; especially the limbs of females, when they are frequently bathed with cold water, emit such a sweet, milky aroma. One observes this when matters of courtesy brings one in contact with such a lady—I mean, when he kisses the hand or lips of such a lady.

Priessnitz is opposed to salt water. Salt water has not the pure quality of the penetration and solution of bodies, but more of corrosion, by means of its fine acrid and salty properties, and, consequently, is incapable of effecting a true radical cure. For, in and after the salt-water bath, the body reacts, not only against the dissolvent power, but also against the penetration of salty and acrid substance. Since a greater part of its energy must be directed against this latter, it cannot direct its undivided strength against its old deep-lodged matters of disease. This salt water, and the mineral spring, belong quite in the category of medicine, because all these unclean waters possess constituents which operate solely by their medicinal effect.

Therefore, the following remarks are more applicable to lake and river bathing than to sea bathing.

These baths, as they have hitherto been used, cannot possibly be of any considerable efficiency. Compared with a systematic water-treatment, their curative effect is as insignificant, as it is excellent in comparison with the effect of medicine.

The season fixed upon for their employment is generally unsuitable; the water, in the months of July and August, is so warm, that their otherwise good effects are, on this account, much diminished. Let him choose these months, who will bathe only for the sake of pleasure; but he who will fish from the sea the delicious pearl of health, should select that time of the year in which the water ranges from 55° to 75° Fahrenheit—the months of April, May, and June—still better, from the middle of August to October and November. But then the duration of the bath must not exceed fifteen minutes—for most patients, not one minute. They must always bathe with the skin warm, or in a slight perspiration.

In the morning take a full bath immediately on coming from bed, while the skin still retains the warmth of the bed; indeed, it is then necessary that the bath be but a few steps distant from the house. If not, one must erect a wooden bathing hut on the strand or shore, and there sweat or heat up in blankets before bathing.

Also, before noon, take a sitz or foot-bath, after which take a walk before dinner. The sitz bath may be taken by all that suffer from dyspepsia, constipation, or nervous affections.

For the afternoon, I would propose a new kind of bath—walking half-baths—that is, in this manner, that the patient must walk from five to ten minutes in the sea, with half of his body immersed in water. The upper part of the body must be so covered, that it is neither too cold nor too hot; that is, it must not perspire. Such a bath would be especially serviceable in drawing congestions from the head and breast. Its first effect would be the contrary; and for this reason, those who are subject thereto, or afflicted therewith, must wet their head and breast with water on going into it. These baths would be particularly effective in conducting the energy, warmth, the matters of disease, and the critical exanthema, from the nobler parts to the legs; they would also particularly benefit those having lame or stiff limbs and joints, or withered calves of the legs.

My above-mentioned conclusions, taken from baths in natural life, led me to the idea of these walking half-baths.

In making use of all local baths, one should consider well the oft-mentioned principle, and, consequently, never take a local bath without combining it with a daily general bath. Under this latter condition, a daily sitz-bath is of inestimable value to sedentary persons who are afflicted with constipation and piles. Priessnitz has restored a great many of these sufferers; all, when they left Graefenberg, took with them their syringe, and respected it as their protective patron. In injections, only cold and tepid water is to be used, and never warm water; their temperature should vary from 55° to 72° Fahrenheit

Woman: Her Education and Influence: With a General Introduction. By Mrs. C. M. Kirkland. With thirteen portraits of distinguished Women. Suitable for a present. 40 cents.

Chemistry Applied to Physiology, Agriculture, AND COMMERCE. By Professor Liebig. A good work. With Additions, by Dr. John Gardner. Large octavo. Best Edition. 20 cents.

Fascination, or the Philosophy of Charming (Magnetism). Illustrating the Principles of Life in Connection with Spirit and Matter. Physiologically considered. Illustrated. 10,000 copies sold. Price, 40 cents.

American Phrenological Journal and Miscellany; Devoted to Phrenology, Physiology, Magnetism, Self-Improvement, and all the reforms of the age. Terms, in advance, $1 00 a year.

Water-Cure Journal and Herald of Reforms: Devoted to Hydropathy and Medical Reform. Terms, in advance, $1 a-year.

Water-Cure in Every Known Disease. By J. H. Rausse. Translated, by C. H. Meeker, M.D., from the German. 50 cents.

The Water-Cure Manual. A popular work on Hydropathy. By Joel Shew, M.D. Every family should have a copy. It contains full directions for the application of water in various diseases. 50 cents.

Lectures on the Philosophy of Mesmerism and CLAIRVOYANCE. With instruction in its process and practical application. Recently republished in London. 25 cents.

Elements of Animal Magnetism: or Process and Practical Application for relieving Human Suffering. 12½ cents.

A Sober and Temperate Life: With Notes and Illustrations, by John Burdell, Dentist. 500,000 copies have been sold. 25 cents.

The Teeth: Their Structure, Disease and Management, with the Causes of Early Decay. With directions for their preservation. By John Burdell, Dental Surgeon. Extensively illustrated. 12½ cents.

The Parents' Guide for the Transmission of Desired Qualities to Offspring, and Childbirth made Easy. By Mrs. Pendleton. The importance of this work is beyond description. 50 cents.

Popular Phrenology, Exhibiting the Phrenological Admeasurement of above fifty distinguished personages. By F. Coombs, Phrenologist. Illustrated with numerous engravings. 25 cents.

The Phrenological Bust, Designed especially for Learners; showing the exact Location of all the Organs of the Brain fully developed. $1 25. ☞ It may be sent by express, or as freight, not by mail.

Natural Laws of Man, Physiologically Con-SIDERED. By Dr. Spurzheim. A work of great merit—only 25 cents.

A Defence of Phrenology. By Dr. Boardman. The arguments of the author are irresistible and convincing. A good work for sceptics and unbelievers. It will overthrow all objections. 50 cents.

Synopsis of Phrenology: A Chart, for recording various Developments: Designed for the Use of Practical Phrenologists. 170,000 copies have been sold. Amply illustrated. 6 1-4 cents.

Temperance and Tight-Lacing: Founded on the Laws of Life, as developed by the Sciences of Phrenology and Physiology. Showing the evil effects of stimulants and tight-lacing. Illustrated. 12½ cents.

Familiar Lessons on Phrenology and Physi-OLOGY: Designed for the Use of Children and Youth, in Schools and Families. Illustrated with sixty-five Engravings. 75 cents.
The price of Physiology, cheap edition, is 25 cents; Phrenology, do., 50 cents.

Familiar Lessons on Astronomy; Do. With Portraits of distinguished Astronomers. Beautifully illustrated by Howland. It should be presented to every youth. Price, only 40 cents.

Marriage: its History and Philosophy; with a Phrenological and Physiological Exposition of the Functions and Qualifications for Happy Marriages. Illustrated. 37½ cents.

Symbolical Head and Phrenological Chart in Map Form; Designed to convey at one view the natural Language of each Organ of the Brain. It is suitable for framing. 25 cents.

The Phrenological Guide; Designed for the Use of Students of their own characters. Containing the first principles of the science. Illustrated with thirty-five Engravings—only 12½ cents.

Synopsis of Phrenology and Physiology: Comprising a condensed Description of the Body and Mind. Illustrated with Engravings. 12½ cents.

The Phrenological and Physiological Alma-NAC, published annually—containing illustrated Descriptions of many of the most distinguished Characters living. Yearly sales, 200,000 copies. Price, per dozen, 50 cents; single copies, 6 1-4 cents.

The Principles of Physiology Applied to the Improvement of Physical and Mental Education. By Andrew Combe, M.D. With Notes and Observations, by O. S. Fowler. 50 cents.

Infancy: or the Physiological and Moral Management of Children. By Andrew Combe, M.D.; with Notes and a Supplement, by Dr. John Bell. Fathers and mothers, read this book. Illustrated. 50 cents.

The Constitution of Man, Considered in Relation to External Objects, with a portrait of the Author, George Combe. A new, revised, enlarged, and illustrated edition. This is the only authorized American edition. No individual should be without it. 50 cents.

Education, Founded on the Nature of Man: Containing an illustrated description of the Temperaments, and a brief Analysis of all the Phrenological Organs. An excellent work. 50 cents.

Human Rights, and their Political Guaran-TIES: Founded on the Moral and Intellectual Laws of our Being. Enlarged edition. *By* E. P. Hurlbut, Judge of Supreme Court, New York. 50 cents.

www.ingramcontent.com/pod-product-compliance
Lightning Source LLC
LaVergne TN
LVHW010215110826
845151LV00004B/1089